Other Books by Steven Waterhouse

Not By Bread Alone; An Outlined Guide to Bible Doctrine

Blessed Assurance; A Defense of the Doctrine of Eternal Security

What Must I Do To Be Saved?
The Bible's Definition of Saving Faith

Life's Tough Questions

Outside the Heavenly City; Abortion in Rome and the Early Church's Response

Holy Matrimony: The Image of God in the Family

Depression Recovery: According to the Bible

Suffering: Why Would a Good God Allow Suffering & Pain?

Bible Truths When Confronting Death

A Biblical Look at Unborn Children

Bible Counsel for Raising Children

Jesus and History: How We Know His Life and Claims

Husband and Wife: The Imitation of Christ

Messianic Prophecy: Confirmation That The Bible is True

Jesus, Miracles and History

NOTE: All are available for free download at
www.webtheology.com.

Strength For His People

A Ministry for Families of the Mentally Ill

Dr. Steven Waterhouse
Th. M., D. Min.

First edition 1994
Reprint 2020 (New Cover)
Reprint 2021 (New Cover)

Westcliff Press
P.O. Box 1521, Amarillo TX 79105

Dear Friends of the Mentally Ill,

Westcliff Bible Church has a genuine concern for your needs and desires to serve the Lord Jesus Christ through ministering to you.

We have reserved a copyright, however, you have permission to duplicate any material you find beneficial. We only request that distribution be on a non-profit basis.

The primary contribution in *Strength For His People* comes from the application of the Bible to the specific questions and needs among Christian families of the mentally ill. Medical research is necessary, but not sufficient, to cope with human problems. We believe you will find the Bible gives wise counsel for handling hardships.

Many readers ask about my brother, Mark Waterhouse. He has made great improvement on clozapine and takes pleasure that his adversity will help others.

Strength For His People or any other of Dr. Waterhouse's writings may be obtained from Westcliff Press, (806) 359-6362; by fax (806) 359-6882; email, westcliff@amaonline.com; or at www.webtheology.com. We encourage local AMI affiliates to secure copies for library donations or to give to interested clergy, counselors, or chaplains.

In God's service,

Pastor Steven Waterhouse, Th.M., D.Min.
Westcliff Bible Church
P.O. Box 1521, Amarillo TX 79105

Dedication

This book is dedicated to Mark Waterhouse
and to our parents, Mr. and Mrs. William Waterhouse
of Athens, Michigan. If I can not cure you, my dear brother,
I will try to use your sufferings to bring hope to hurting
families and enlightenment to neglectful churches.

Table of Contents

Chapter One

The Trouble I've Seen: At Home and in the Church

My beloved younger brother awoke me with a terrifying shriek. I jumped from bed and rushed to see him "fighting" with non-existent people. He grabbed a praying hands plaque and smashed it into the wall. He ripped a Bible with great zeal. He tore the light fixture from the ceiling and pulled the wires through the cracking plaster. "What's wrong?", I pleaded. "Nothing...go back to sleep," Mark replied in a calm manner.

I could neither sleep nor go back to life as usual. My brother suffers from schizophrenia. Over time he has taken the furniture to the front lawn to burn it and pushed our mother through a screen door. One time we stopped at a red light, and he fled from the car. He has a compulsion to drink so much liquid that it endangers his life by washing out essential minerals from his system. He was one of only three people in a western Michigan mental hospital to have a full time guard. Someone had to keep him from sinks, showers and toilets. He might have killed himself by drinking water. Mark also tortures himself by the thought that he murdered someone. No amount of rational evidence, including letters from a kind district judge, persuades him otherwise. Of all his behavior and actions, I had the most trouble with Mark's attempt at self-castration. He spent five days healing in the hospital. He hurt most, but he was not the only one with pain.

Families suffer with their loved ones. They typically suffer without much professional help, medical or ministerial. In most cases they rally with deep dedication and courage. Maryellen Walsh describes a typical reaction, "Hell or high water, in sickness and in more sickness, love continues to rise within the family ..."[1] My family has done well considering the severity with which schizophrenia ravages relationships. However, I was astounded at the basic lack of

---

[1]Maryellen Walsh, *Schizophrenia: Straight Talk for Family and Friends*, reprint ed. (New York: Warner Books, Inc., 1985), 30.

professional support for families of people with schizophrenia. I could forgive the psychiatric community for not having a complete solution for mental illness. They are not superhuman. Yet, why was there so little literature for the relatives? Why so little time for consultation? Could not professionals see the obvious? Families suffer too!

Fortunately, health care professionals have begun to realize the needs of such families. Surveys taken in 1982 yielded a 74% dissatisfaction rate with services to the families of those with mental illness while only 8% responded with confidence in mental health professionals.[2] The 80's saw the publication of several wonderful books for families who have a relative with schizophrenia.[3] Some books are family aids. Others direct institutional program development so that health care professionals can help families.[4] It appears that the days of a Freudian approach to the families of those with schizophrenia will pass away. Instead of falsely blaming relatives for causing schizophrenia, future mental health programs will desire to care for families, as well as, consumers.[5] This is a happy development. Yet, while secular professionals have tried to improve their programs, churches and clergy remain weak in ministry to hurting amilies.[6]

[2]Kayla F. Bernheim and Anthony F. Lehman, *Working with Families of the Mentally Ill* (New York: W.W. Norton and Company, 1985), 14.

[3]I would most highly recommend *Schizophrenia* by Maryellen Walsh and *Surviving Schizophrenia* by E. Fuller Torrey.

[4]The following are major studies done for the purpose of improving services for families: Bernheim, Kayla F. and Anthony F. Lehman, *Working with Families of the Mentally Ill.* New York: W.W. Norton and Company, 1985; Hatfield, Agnes B. *Family Education in Mental Illness.* New York: The Guilford Press, 1990; Hatfield, Agnes B. and Harriet P. Lefley, eds. *Families of the Mentally Ill: Coping and Adaptation.* New York: The Guilford Press, 1987; and Lefley, Harriet P. and Dale L. Johnson. *Families as Allies in the Treatment of the Mentally Ill.* Washington, D.C.: American Psychiatric Press, 1990.

[5]"Consumer" refers to a person who has a mental illness.

[6]A search at a prominent seminary which has an excellent theological library resulted in finding only one book about families of the mentally ill. This single volume was written in 1957 (before deinstitutionalization of consumers from large state mental hospitals) and ironically had the word "discarded" written on the inside. Theological journals contain few articles on families of the mentally ill. The Summer and Fall 1990 issues of *The Journal of Pastoral Care* are pleasant exceptions.

Our church did not know how to minister to my family. Those ignorant of both mental illness and theology tended to blame schizophrenia on sin or bad parenting. Thus, they found it easy to withdraw from our suffering. At a time when we needed Christian support most, we experienced an awkward avoidance. I harbor no bitterness towards them. They reflect a larger culture that is ignorant about schizophrenia and avoids the unknown. Such Christians need to be taught, not condemned. Christian members in the National Alliance for the Mentally Ill (NAMI) should not reject churches but rather, work to improve them. The Waterhouse family's experience represents the typical weakness in clergy/church ministry to families of those with schizophrenia. Dr. Torrey claims that schizophrenia challenges a parent's "theological core."[7] Therefore, one would think a seminary education could include a few lectures on mental illness as part of the pastoral counseling curriculum. Even if medical help for consumers is beyond the scope of pastoral ministry, surely families remain a pastoral responsibility. In my eight years of college and seminary training, there was not a single lecture devoted to mental illness. Such neglect shows up in ministry. In 1983 the California Alliance For the Mentally Ill conducted a survey to determine the source to which families went for help and the value of any help received. Of twelve common sources, clergy ranked last in helpfulness.[8]

In California forty percent of families of the mentally ill go to a minister for help.[9] However, they find little. I believe this must change.

The Scriptures provide many answers to the emotional turmoil experienced by relatives of those with mental illness. Secular books on mental illness describe the pain families endure, but the church could

---

[7]Walsh, *Schizophrenia*, 9.

[8]Ibid., 139.

[9]Ibid. This figure involves only the families. Mentally ill people also typically look to their minister first when searching for help. "Religious organizations in particular... have been the most remiss in service to the mentally ill and their families... Three other studies have shown that between 40-42% of Americans turn to their clergy first when confronted with serious mental health problems. In contrast 25% went to general physicians, 17% to psychiatrists, and only 10% went to mental health facilities..." *NAMI Religious Outreach Network Resource Materials* (Arlington, VA: The National Alliance for the Mentally Ill, n.d.), 3.

actually do a superior job of prescribing answers. Theology can excel psychology in giving a philosophy of suffering. The church should be the ultimate support group. Christianity has a great contribution to make in the area of ministry to families struggling with schizophrenia. Christian workers should learn to apply the Scriptures to the needs of these families. In reality, it may be that families will learn to care for their own spiritual needs first, and then they will teach Christian professionals how to minister to others. Maybe you could explain to your pastor how to minister to relatives of people with mental illness by suggesting educational resources or by encouraging attendance at local Alliance for the Mentally Ill meetings. Most pastors probably did not learn how to minister to families of the mentally ill in seminary. In fact, many have the false impression that mental illness does not even exist, or they believe psychiatry is so hostile to religion that it has no value.

These problems bring us to our next study. Chapter Two will involve issues such as: Does mental illness really exist? What is known about the cause of schizophrenia? Does psychiatry have any value for Christians? In the following chapters we will give much attention to theology. However, misunderstandings about the causes of schizophrenia will lead to terrible misapplication of the Bible. Therefore, even though our ultimate goals are spiritual, we must begin with medical research. You can also use these medical facts to explain your relative's schizophrenia to others.

Questions and Thoughts to Consider from Chapter One

1. How would you have viewed people with schizophrenia before you faced it in your own family? How would most psychiatrists have viewed families as recently as twenty years ago?

2. How were your experiences with your church or minister similar or different from our family's experience?

3. If your experience was unpleasant, do you believe that awkwardness due to ignorance on the part of church members played a larger role than sheer meanness?

4. Would your minister read a Christian book about brain disorders? Will your church library accept such a book? (I would suggest *Counselor's Guide To The Brain And Its Disorders: Knowing the Difference Between Disease and Sin* by Edward T. Welch. This was published by Zondervan in 1991.)

5. How could the Alliance for the Mentally Ill help clergy to understand schizophrenia? How can we influence seminary curriculum?

Chapter 2

Schizophrenia: Causes and Theological Classification

I have delivered a sermon called "Psychiatry: Voodoo or Virtue?" Actually, it is a trick title representing two erroneous extremes. Some Christians can see no good in psychiatry. They regard it as totally "of the devil". Others can see no flaws in psychiatry. They act as if it offers a new priesthood with new answers equal to Scripture. The truth lies in creating a third option: limited value. Psychiatry is not all virtue, but neither is it complete voodoo. Sensible people will recognize psychiatry's limited value. While the psychiatric and psychological professions can be legitimately criticized from a Christian perspective, it does not follow that Christians must reject all truth or all help from this field of learning.[10] Secular mental health experts help us most by describing human problems and treating genuine medical problems.

If you have a loved one in need of psychiatric care, you may feel great uneasiness, especially if your minister disapproves of all secular mental health care. It will help you to understand psychiatry's limited value without having to view psychiatry as a substitute religion with ultimate answers to life.

Secular mental health professionals primarily benefit Christians in the area of medicine. Most Christians grant this principle with medical problems such as cancer, diabetes, or asthma but have more trouble with mental illness. Is there really any valid theological reason that requires the brain to be the only organ immune from disorders? Most Christians would grant a medical basis to mental retardation. We neither blame retardation on bad parenting nor expect the handicapped to overcome their limitations by will power. Likewise, it would be cruel to read a Bible passage to an Alzheimer's victim and command him to

---

[10]Gary Collins, William Kirk Kilpatrick, and Martin and Deidre Bobgan give excellent studies on the conflict between Christianity and psychology. See Collins, Gary. *Can You Trust Psychology?* Downers Grove, IL: Inter-Varsity Press,1988; Kilpatrick, William Kirk. *Psychological Seduction*. Nashville: Thomas Nelson Publishers, 1983; and Bobgan, Martin and Deidre Bobgan. *Psychoheresy*. Santa Barbara, CA: East Gate Publishers, 1987.

snap out of it. Alzheimer's is clearly a medical illness rather than a moral choice. Although researchers do not yet know the exact cause, autopsies coupled recently with brain scans establish that Alzheimer's ravages the brain. Alzheimer's disease leaves a signature that is unmistakable. The brains of victims are packed with two types of abnormalities, called tangles and plaques. Tangles appear as dense, insoluble clots of material inside damaged brain cells, or neurons. Plaques appear on the outside of neurons. They are clumps of special protein intertwined with dead and dying bunches of surrounding nerves. It is not known whether plaques and tangles actually destroy neurons or if they are simply the by-products of Alzheimer's ruinous effects.[11]

Mental illness could have other physiological bases. It would be hard to argue against evidence that "strokes, tumors, malaria, syphilis, poisonings, vitamin deficiencies, hypothyroidism, temporal lobe deficiency, viral infections" and maybe other factors can affect our minds.[12] Even those most opposed to psychology and psychiatry in general should make room for seeing the value of secular help for genuine medical disorders.

Most understand that problems such as mental retardation or Alzheimer's have a biological basis, but some have trouble classifying other mental illnesses such as schizophrenia as medical problems. People have compassion for the young and elderly but often fix blame upon those who develop mental illness in the prime of life.

Often they are blamed for falling victim to an illness that has a clear biological basis. A 1988 survey of Utah residents found widespread prejudice against mental illness. 71% of respondents believed mental illness is due to emotional weakness; 65% believed it is due to bad parenting, 35% felt it

---

[11]Sharon Brownlee, "Alzheimer's: Is There Hope?" *U.S. News and World Report,* 12 August 1991, 42. See also chapters 17 and 18 in Mace, Nancy L., and Peter V. Rabins. *The 36 Hour Day: A Family Guide to Caring For Persons with Alzheimer's Disease.* New York: Warner Books Inc., 1981.

[12]E. Fuller Torrey, *Surviving Schizophrenia: A Family Manual*, rev. ed.(New York: Perennial Library of Harper and Row Publishers, 1988), 338.

is due to sinful behavior; and 43% felt that mentally ill people bring on their own illness.[13]

Christians, including ministers who blame consumers, have probably never researched disorders like schizophrenia. Because the surrounding culture is ignorant of and biased against mental illness, it is easy to absorb that same ignorance and bias. No doubt the tendency of some to attribute all behavioral flaws to a medical condition pushes Christians in the direction of objecting to any behavioral problem having a biological foundation. Christian professionals would object to tracing most teenage disobedience back to genetics. Thus, we can be stubborn about conceding that any unacceptable behavior has a medical origin. My brother's attempt to burn furniture might be evaluated as pure rebellion instead of a medical abnormality. However, secular mental health professionals have amassed credible evidence supporting the classification of schizophrenia as a disorder of the brain. Christians do not need to approve every particular in modern psychology and psychiatry in order to appreciate the value of help for medical problems. Researchers do not have complete answers, but they know enough to classify schizophrenia as a medical disorder instead of a moral deficiency.[14] Reasons for viewing schizophrenia as a medical problem can be classified under studies on families and brain research.

---

[13]"Facts About Mental Illness," (Austin, TX: Texas Alliance for the Mentally Ill, n.d.), 1.

[14]While one might have an opinion about the role of personal sin in a particular incident of sickness, it would be difficult to prove it categorically or generalize about a theology of mental illness. The Bible allows many other reasons God might permit affliction. Most do not involve personal sin. Also, sins and flaws existing in every person could tentatively be viewed as the theological cause for an individual's sickness. However, there will be much conjecture when we attempt to explain another person's sickness. God may directly give an individual a conviction that sin brought on a sickness, but it is not possible to become the Holy Spirit for another person and to assess God's reason for allowing his sickness. In this regard mental illness would be like any other disease, except a mentally ill person might have trouble with an objective assessment of sin or the lack of it in his life. My poor brother thinks he's a murderer!

Two things are clear: A mentally ill person may have sinned less than a mentally healthy person; and once mental illness begins, it has a definite medical aspect. Both truths demand that Christians approach persons with mental illness in humility and mercy.

Family Studies

Although researchers admit they do not have the ultimate answers to the causes of schizophrenia, they do have some firm conclusions. One major view argues for multiple factors with an emphasis upon a genetic predisposition toward the disorder that is perhaps triggered by stress.[15] That stress alone does not cause schizophrenia is supported by the fact that few diagnoses of schizophrenia resulted from the Normandy invasion.[16] A person must have a genetic vulnerability to schizophrenia before any other factors push him over the threshold into manifestations of schizophrenia. Thus, heredity may not be the only factor, but it is a main one. Genes alone are not sufficient to explain schizophrenia, but they are necessary. Psychiatrists draw these conclusions based upon observations of family risk, studies of adopted children, and studies of identical twins.

Family Risk

While the risk for a typical American of getting schizophrenia is 1 out of 100, the risk for relatives of those with schizophrenia increases. The following chart is adapted from Dr. Irving I. Gottesman's book *Schizophrenia Genesis.*[17]

Relationship to Consumer	Risk
General population	1%
First cousins	2%
Uncles/Aunts	2%
Nephews/Nieces	4%
Grandchildren	5%

---

[15]Nancy C. Andreasen, *The Broken Brain: The Biological Revolution in Psychiatry* (New York: Harper and Row, 1984), 222; and Irving I. Gottesman, *Schizophrenia Genesis: The Origins of Madness* (New York: W.H. Freeman and Company, 1991), 82,90-93.

[16]Ibid., 152.

[17]Ibid., 96. For a second chart, please consult Maryellen Walsh, *Schizophrenia: Straight Talk for Family and Friends*, reprint ed. (New York: Warner Books, Inc., 1985), 69.

Half-brother/sister	6%
Children	13%
Brother or Sister	9%
Fraternal twins	17%
Identical twins	48%
Children with both parents having schizophrenia	46%

Such evidence suggests "the magnitude of the increased risk varies with the amount of gene sharing and not with the amount of experience sharing."[18] Heredity alone may not predestine one to schizophrenia, but it gives a strong influence.[19] Those who would argue that the above statistics arise from a shared environment in the home and not shared genes must do so against repeated studies on children of persons with schizophrenia who have been adopted and raised without contact with their biological parents. When such children develop schizophrenia, it must come from shared genetic vulnerability with their biological parents rather than a shared environment with them.

Adoption Studies

We will consider cumulative evidence for a genetic predisposition to schizophrenia by looking at three studies in widely separate regions: Oregon, Denmark, and Israel.

Leonard Heston in 1966 studied grown children who had been born to mothers in Oregon state mental hospitals and placed either in orphanages or with paternal relatives. The result was that 16.6% of the offspring had developed schizophrenia.[20] That figure is even higher than one that includes children raised by a parent with schizophrenia (see previous chart). It appears that genetics influenced the outcome

---

[18]Gottesman, *Schizophrenia Genesis*, 97.

[19]The above statistics do not present evidence for a single gene being the culprit. If that were the case, one would expect numbers such as 50% or 25%. Dr. Gottesman uses the term "polygenic" throughout his book meaning a whole group of unfortunate genes causes a disposition to schizophrenia. On page 87 he lists diseases with similar patterns including diabetes, coronary heart disease, and Alzheimer's disease.

[20]Ibid., 136-137.

regardless of who raised the children. Additional adoption studies confirm a role for heredity in the origin of schizophrenia.

Denmark keeps excellent records on its citizens. Therefore, researchers could track the children whose biological parents had schizophrenia but whose adoptive parents did not. Dr. E. Fuller Torrey summarizes the results: The children were followed up after they had become adults, and it was found that children of schizophrenic parents retained their increased predisposition toward developing the disease despite the fact that they had been raised by non-schizophrenic parents.[21]

The risk for getting schizophrenia tended to be the same for these children regardless of whether they lived with a biological parent who had schizophrenia or with adopted parents. Thus, studies in Denmark confirm that genetic factors are necessary to explain the origin of schizophrenia. Finally, adoption studies from Israel give fascinating results. In 1965 the National Institute of Mental Health (NIMH) and Israeli researchers began a study. Part of that study involved 50 children who each had one parent with schizophrenia. Half of the group were raised by parents at home. The other 25 were raised on a kibbutz, an Israeli communal settlement. The test's hypotheses were that removal of children from a parent with schizophrenia might prevent the disorder and that professional caregivers in the commune could reduce the risk for schizophrenia. The results by 1981 had proved otherwise.

Of the 23 kibbutz-reared children of schizophrenics found in the follow-up study, a total of 16, or 70% showed signs of mental illness, while only 29% of those raised at home were assigned a DSM III diagnoses.[22]

---

[21]E. Fuller Torrey, *Surviving Schizophrenia: A Family Manual*, Rev. ed. (New York: Harper and Row, 1988), 145.

[22]Harriet P.Lefley, "Culture and Mental Illness: The Family Role," in *Families of the Mentally Ill: Coping and Adaptation*, edited by Agnes B. Hatfield and Harriet P. Lefley (New York: The Guilford Press, 1987), 36. She also writes about Israeli Studies in Harriet P. Lefley, "Research Directions for a New Conceptualization of Families," in *Families as Allies in the Treatment of the Mentally Ill*, edited by Harriet P.Lefley and Dale C. Johnson (Washington, DC: American Psychiatric Press, 1990), 144.

Score one for motherhood! Also, consider the cumulative evidence from adoption studies that shared genes, as opposed to shared environment, create the tendency toward schizophrenia.

Statistics on family risk and adoption studies both argue that schizophrenia is largely a medical problem. A third area of family research involves that favorite area for testing, studies on twins.

Twin Studies

When one identical twin has schizophrenia, the other will also have it approximately 50% of the time.[23] If genetics were the only factor in schizophrenia, then both twins would always develop schizophrenia. As we said earlier, heredity must be a factor to create a predisposition to schizophrenia, but other factors act as a trigger when a person has the unlucky genetic weakness.[24]

Although studies of identical twins show other factors at work, they also show that risks increase as one shares more genetic material with a mentally ill relative. Identical twins have identical genes and also comprise the highest risk category on the chart on page 24.The most enlightening studies on identical twins concern their offspring. In situations where one identical twin has schizophrenia but the other does not, the offspring of the healthy twin has the same risk for schizophrenia as the offspring of his sibling. Gottesman lists the risks to children of "healthy" twins at 17.4% and the risks to children of twins with schizophrenia at 16.8%.[25] This means that shared genes with an uncle or aunt contribute towards schizophrenia whereas parenting by one with schizophrenia does not increase the risk.

Again, the evidence from twin studies, adoption studies, and general family studies point to schizophrenia being a disorder largely

---

[23]Nancy C. Andreasen, *The Broken Brain*, 229.

[24]Gottesman says, "When human geneticists estimate the magnitude of genetic factors contributing to the liability for developing schizophrenia, they obtain a value of about 70% for that statistic termed *heritability*." Gottesman, *Schizophrenia Genesis*, 163.

[25]Ibid., 123-125.

caused by a genetic predisposition. Therefore, it appears safe to conclude that schizophrenia is fundamentally an underlying medical problem. It is also safe to expect that brain research will eventually provide strong evidence that schizophrenia is a medical problem. The 1980's saw the development of technologies that enabled physicians to look inside the brain. While objective researchers cannot yet give absolute determinations about the causes of schizophrenia, conclusions about the disorder will never be the same.

Brain Research

An involved discussion on brain research would detract from our overall purpose of developing a theological view of schizophrenia. For our purposes we only need to consider whether brain research contributes to the position that schizophrenia involves medical problems. Those with deeper interest should read Dr. Nancy Andreasen's book, *The Broken Brain,* or chapter six in Dr. E. Fuller Torrey's *Surviving Schizophrenia: A Family Manual.* The National Alliance for the Mentally Ill distributes a Cable News Network (CNN) video with a segment of the broadcast "News From Medicine." Its second segment also gives helpful information about brain research.[26]

Researchers have been interested in structural differences between the brains of people with schizophrenia and those without the disorder. Some consumers definitely have enlarged cavities called ventricles.[27] This abnormality seems to indicate a "shrinkage of the brain because neurons have died."[28] However, most people with schizophrenia do not have enlarged ventricles. Estimates of those who do range from 10% to 50%.[29] This means physicians have not been able to create a test that

---

[26]Christians will particularly enjoy the first segment as it features former Green Bay Packer, Lionel Aldridge, who is a Christian who has schizophrenia. NAMI publishes a book list which will give the most recent sources for medical research.

[27]Ventricles contain cerebrospinal fluid. There are four of them. For a survey of recent studies about the relationship between brain ana-tomy/chemistry and schizophrenia see Gershon, Elliot S. and Ronald O. Rieder. "Major Disorders of the Mind and Brain." *Scientific American* 267 (September 1992): 126-133.

[28]Andreasen, *The Broken Brain*, 225.

[29]Ibid., 226.

precisely indicates schizophrenia by looking for enlarged ventricles. Other studies that receive great attention include the limbic system and tests on cerebral blood flow.[30]

Brain chemistry is a second area of brain research that makes psychiatrists think in terms of biological causes for schizophrenia. Many theories exist about chemical neurotransmitters or the parts of the brain that receive these chemicals.[31]

Leading authorities admit they have much more work to do and at present have tantalizing leads as opposed to solid conclusions. However, they will assert that "a consistent trend appears."[32] Perhaps at a time in the near future, brain research will solve some of the mysteries of schizophrenia. In the meantime, how do these studies bear on the issue of the origin of schizophrenia?

Those who defend a pure family causation view (or believe sin is the only factor in "madness") will criticize the findings of brain research because there has not yet been found a common anatomical or chemical problem in all people with schizophrenia. They might further object that structural differences such as enlarged ventricles are the result rather than the cause of schizophrenia.

However, many experts believe that schizophrenia is really a number of related disorders with multiple causes. Future research may use differences in brain structure or chemistry to *classify different kinds of schizophrenia* and their causes.[33] We do not yet have definite answers, but focus on the above mentioned "trends" may well detect a

---

[30]CNN's "News From Medicine, Peace of Mind" video enables the public to view a cerebral blood flow test and shows that some people with schizophrenia have differences from healthy people in brain structure or function. See also Torrey, *Surviving Schizophrenia,* 134 and 139; Andreasen, *The Broken Brain,* 103.

[31]Andreasen, *The Broken Brain,* 209; Torrey, *Surviving Schizophrenia,* 134-135; Gottesman, *Schizophenia Genesis,* 238.

[32]Ibid.

[33]Experts assume there is more than one kind of schizophrenia and will use this assumption to classify differences they see in brain research. Andreasen, *Broken Brain,* 222; Gottesman, *Schizophrenia Genesis,* 231.

group of related disorders with slightly different causes. It is true that brain research alone has not yet given the definitive origin of schizophrenia, but the evidence which does exist gives no comfort to those who still want to insist medical problems have nothing to do with the disorder. Some people with schizophrenia do have physical abnormalities in their brains. Eventually, medical experts may be able to show that all of them do. Christian psychologist and seminary instructor, Edward T. Welch, writes of this probable outcome of further brain research.

> Yet, we should recognize that Christians have no ax to grind with a biased interpretation of the data. recognize that evidence of subtle physical differences in those with schizophrenic symptoms as compared to those without will probably emerge. If, over the next decade, there is medical research that demonstrates unmistakable differences between brains of schizophrenics and nonschizophrenics, these data should be heralded as potentially valuable and consistent with a theory of schizophrenia that is Biblically permissible. [34]

I hope that information given to this point has made credible the idea that psychiatry is not complete voodoo. Yes, psychiatry does have its flaws, especially from a Christian perspective; but its primary value lies in giving help for genuine medical problems that affect behavior. There is substantial evidence from family studies and potentially new evidence from brain research to conclude that biological weakness plays a dominant role in causing schizophrenia. Even if we do not have complete answers, we know enough to prove that Christians should respond to consumers and their families with empathy and compassion and not with blame and avoidance. Theologians, ministers, and church members must understand a human problem accurately before applying the Bible to it. Failures to understand medical problems can lead to blunders in ministry. British clergy in the 19th century asserted that cholera epidemics were a sign of God's judgment against the sins of lower social classes.[35] Their theological mistake was a failure to

---

[34]Edward T. Welch, *Counselor's Guide To The Brain and its Disorders: Knowing the Difference Between Disease and Sin* (Grand Rapids: Zon-dervan Publishing House, 1991), 231.

[35]Ibid., 16.

appreciate the fact that the Bible gives over a dozen reasons for suffering other than punishment (see Chapter Five for a study on the theology of suffering). Another great mistake lay in a misunderstanding of the problem. People in 19th century England sinned, but cholera is spread by bacteria. Through ignorance of medicine, clergy and church members were misapplying the Bible and harming innocent people in the process. There is a danger of doing the same thing with schizophrenia.

As a Christian and as one trained in Biblical research, I believe the Scriptures have much wisdom for families of the mentally ill. When Christian leaders realize the true nature of schizophrenia, they will have no trouble developing ministries to help both families and consumers. Our generation is no time for churches to be ignorant of medicine.[36]

With the conclusion that schizophrenia is largely, but not totally, a medical problem, we will now turn to a theological classification of the disorder. How can we integrate our understanding of schizophrenia into a Biblical system? This topic will also allow us to return to the role of stress in triggering, but not causing, schizophrenia.

---

[36]I have been hard on the failures of the church in order to provoke changes. However, to be fair there have been equal failures in the secular psychiatric/psychological communities and the general public. These should be at least as humble as the clergy relative to past attitudes toward families or theories about them. I agree with the authors who wrote:

"Church groups are often misunderstood by society as a whole. Mental health workers also harbor negative beliefs about the church as rejecting of the mentally ill, and about church persons as rigid, moralistic, and naive, if not superstitious in their beliefs. The historical misconceptions have persisted far too long. The truth of the matter is that church members have probably been no more or less mistaken in their attitudes and beliefs about mental illness than the general public and that, if anything, church persons have been more predisposed to respond to a call for assistance given the opportunity and some clear idea of the tasks to be done. The long and well-documented history of the church's provision of care and protection for the homeless and helpless serves as ample evidence here."

Richard C. Erickson, David Cutler, Victoria Brannan Cowell, and George E. Dobler, "Serving the Needs of Persons with Chronic Mental Illness, A Neglected Ministry" *The Journal of Pastoral Care* XLIV, No.2 (Summer 1990): 158.

A Theological Classification of Schizophrenia

Now we must try to blend medical evidence with theological evidence. First, we will look at Bible texts that seem to involve mental illness. (For the present we will exclude the issue of demons until Chapter Six.) Then we will examine a theological classification that best incorporates mental illness. We will also consider some suggestions for attitudes towards fellow believers who have mental illnesses. Finally, we will consider the topic of wrongdoing by those with schizophrenia.

Biblical texts on mental illness

Although Scriptures do not present indisputable examples of schizophrenia, some passages reveal that ancient people were acquainted with mental illness in general. Several texts give misdiagnoses by those who wished to discredit another person. At an early point in His ministry, Jesus' relatives "went to take charge of Him, for they said, 'He is out of His mind '" (Mark 3:21 NIV). Festus, the Roman governor of Judea, mentioned insanity in a trial with the Apostle Paul.

> •And while Paul was saying this in his defense, Festus said in a loud voice, "Paul, you are out of your mind! Your great learning is driving you mad." But Paul said, "I am not out of my mind, most excellent Festus, but I utter words of sober truth. For the king knows about these matters, and I speak to him also with confidence, since I am persuaded that none of these things escape his notice; for this has not been done in a corner" (Acts 26:24-25).

Israelite King David pretended to have a mental illness in order to escape a dangerous situation. He apparently felt that the Philistines would be afraid of a mentally ill person and leave him alone.

> • And David took these words to heart, and greatly feared Achish king of Gath. So he disguised his sanity before them, and acted insanely in their hands, and scribbled on the doors of

the gate, and let his saliva run down into his beard. Then Achish said to his servants, "Behold, you see the man behaving as a madman. Why do you bring him to me? Do I lack madmen, that you have brought this one to act the madman in my presence? Shall this one come into my house?" (1 Samuel. 21:12-15)

These texts show that the ancient world was aware of some type of mental illness, but they do not give enough information to build any sort of theology of mental illness. Two additional Old Testament texts are more important.

The book of Daniel teaches that the Babylonian emperor, Nebuchadnezzar, lost his sanity because God was tired of the king's deep and rebellious arrogance. For a time Nebuchadnezzar wandered in isolated places in a disheveled condition eating grass.

- All this happened to Nebuchadnezzer the king. Twelve months later he was walking on the roof of the royal palace of Babylon. The king reflected and said, "Is this not Babylon the great, which I myself have built as a royal residence by the might of my power and for the glory of my majesty?" While the word was in the king's mouth, a voice came from heaven, saying, "King Nebuchadnezzer, to you it is declared: sovereignty has been removed from you, and you will be driven away from mankind, and your dwelling place will be with the beasts of the field. You will be given grass to eat like cattle, and seven periods of time will pass over you, until you recognize that the Most High is ruler over the realm of mankind, and bestows it on whomever He wishes." Immediately the word concerning Nebuchadnezzar was fulfilled; and he was driven away from mankind and began eating grass like cattle, and his body was drenched with the dew of heaven, until his hair had grown like eagles' feathers and his nails like birds' claws. But at the end of that period I, Nebuchadnezzar, raised my eyes toward heaven, and my reason returned to me, and I blessed the Most High and praised and honored Him who lives forever; For His dominion is an everlasting dominion, and His kingdom endures from generation to generation (Daniel 4:28-34).

Fragmentary lines from a tablet in the British Museum (BM 34113) can be interpreted to confirm Nebuchadnezzar's odd behavior:

> [Nebu]chadnezzar considered... his life to be of no value to him.... He gives an entirely different order.... He does not show love to son and daughter.... family and clan do not exist.... He weeps bitterly to Marduk, the great god....[37]

These lines support the Biblical account. King Nebuchadnezzar acted strangely, gave contradictory orders, lost his desire to live, and neglected his family, religion, and empire.

Nebuchadnezzar is a definite Biblical example of some kind of mental illness, although a specific diagnosis is not possible. Here is an example where God judged a ruler by allowing a mental illness. However, it would not be right to generalize his case to all persons with mental illness. The entire book of Job teaches that suffering *can be, but need not be*, a result of sin. The Lord Jesus rebuked his disciples for thinking all affliction arises from sin and taught that others fall into the category of no-fault suffering (see John 9:1-3). Thus, Nebuchadnezzar's example should be included within our thinking but cannot be used to extrapolate a universal truth for all other cases of mental illness. In some cases God allowed (I would not say caused) a mental illness to correct a sin. In other cases the mental illness has to do with many other reasons God allows suffering as explained in Chapter Five. In these ways mental illness would be theologically the same as other sicknesses. The same point will be true for the next Scripture passage in Deut. 28, but Deut. 28 also gives an important contribution by listing insanity in a group of definite medical problems. The LORD will smite you with the boils of Egypt and with tumors and with the scab and with the itch, from which you cannot be healed. The LORD

---

[37]Siegfried Horn, "What is New in Biblical Archeology?," *Ministry*, Supplement. Siegfried Horn, Ph.D. is dean and professor of archeology and history of antiquity, emeritus, at Andrews University in Berrien Springs, Michigan.

will smite you with madness and with blindness and with bewilderment of heart (Deut. 28:27-28).[38]

Notice the items in this list that do not pertain to psychological problems: boils, tumors, festering sores, skin diseases (the itch) and blindness. These are medical problems. The text allows the interpretation that "madness" also belongs in a list of medical problems.

God might permit tumors to grow in order to correct a sin problem, or He might allow a tumor for a reason that has nothing to do with sin. Either way, a tumor is a medical problem with a physiological cause and needs medical treatment. Even if we could somehow prove that God permitted a specific tumor to correct sin, the fact remains that having the tumor is not the sin. Furthermore, it would be best to view the cause of the tumor as medical with God using a medical problem to correct a spiritual one. I believe Christians should view schizophrenia as they would tumors or any other illness.

Christianity does not need to construct an entirely new model for ministry to those with schizophrenia or their families. Ministry to them should generally correspond to ministry to those with other illnesses. To make the point, let us return to the comparison with tumors. How would a church minister to a member with a serious tumor and his or her family?

If a known wrong does exist, then a pastor should encourage its confession to God (see 1 John 1:9) with the assurance of a complete forgiveness for those who have trusted in Christ as Savior. However, if an afflicted person knows of no unrepented sin, there is no need whatsoever to probe any further with the presupposition that there must be spiritual problems at the root of the disease. There does not have to be any spiritual problem, and it would be most cruel to suggest family failures created their relative's suffering. Someone -it need not be clergy- should teach the patient and family about the many other Biblical reasons God might allow for suffering in a believer's life and encourage them to ask God for wisdom as to which truths apply to their

[38]It would be a mistake to apply warnings given to Israel to God's people in the Church because Israel and the Church are two distinct works of God.

case of having a tumor (James 1:5). The congregation should minister to the family in practical ways giving a network of support and providing respite care if needed. Transfer the approach Christians should take to families of tumor patients to relatives of those with schizophrenia, and it will give basic wisdom about Christian responsibility to them.

The texts in this section contain virtually all of the direct information that the Bible gives on mental illness. There is additional value in considering an overall theological classification that best encompasses schizophrenia.

Human weakness [39]

Having schizophrenia is no more a sin than having cancer. Even if sin is a triggering factor in some cases, the underlying cause is still a genetic weakness towards schizophrenia. Categorizing schizophrenia as a weakness rather than a sin has great implications for attitudes toward those who profess faith in Jesus Christ and suffer with schizophrenia.

Attitudes Toward Christians with Schizophrenia

My brother Mark trusted in Christ as Savior at an early age. His schizophrenia created great weakness and spiritual struggles of the intensity most will never know. Strange voices tell him to commit horrible crimes. He fights back to resist these temptations and has so far fought a good fight. Certainly, Christians with schizophrenia have ac-countability before the Lord Jesus Christ for their moral behavior. They still have responsibility and the capability for ethical behavior. They still have the spiritual capacity for closeness to Christ.[40] Christian living is not impossible for them, but it is more difficult. They have weaknesses that can make it harder to resist anger or fear or the temptation to lie or steal. Dr. Edward Welch gives an insightful note to summarize the higher calling to believers who are mentally ill.

---

[39]Dr. Welch influenced some of my thinking here.

[40]While conducting chapel services for the Panhandle Alliance for the Mentally Ill, I observed that many of the consumers have a high de-gree of dedication to the Lord Jesus Christ.

Therefore, it is possible to have schizophrenic symptoms but have neither a specific, sinful origin to them nor a sinful response. It is as if the Bible says, "In your madness, sin not."[41]

Christians who do not share these infirmities should learn to appreciate the deep spiritual conflicts within those who suffer from schizophrenia. They should consider that God may someday give great honor to believers with brain disorders who fought and won victories over their infirmities. Everyone who trusts Christ as Savior ends in heaven. It is possible that Mark will have a greater honor there than his big brother.

Schizophrenia and sinless perfection

Having schizophrenia is not a sin, and the disorder is not caused by sinning. Many very wicked people never develop schizophrenia because they do not have a biological predisposition to it. Sin alone will not cause schizophrenia. Nevertheless, after these conclusions we must still come back to the Biblical assertion that "all have sinned" (Romans 3:23). To say that genuine mental illness is not a sin is not the same as saying people with mental illness have attained sinless perfection. To say that families do not cause schizophrenia is not the same as saying families stand morally faultless. Contrary to impressions in some circles, both families and consumers are very much fallible; and failure to obtain forgiveness for sin from Christ will only make our lives far worse. Although schizophrenia is not caused by sin, in some cases sinful activity may have led to intense stress that in turn triggered schizophrenia. Earlier we stated that some believe stress can trigger schizophrenic symptoms in those who have a genetic weakness. Some of the stressors that push a person over the threshold into schizophrenia involve activities that the Bible would classify as wrong such as drug abuse or cult involvement.[42] It is not that sin alone can trigger initial schizophrenic symptoms, but rather that stress caused by sin can bring on schizophrenia in those predisposed to it. The good news about sin is that God promises to forgive those who have trusted in Christ. Stress can also arise from being a victim of the wrongdoing of others. In

---

[41]Welch, *Counselors Guide to the Brain*, 237.

[42]Gottesman, *Schizophrenia Genesis*, 204.

addition, stresses unrelated to any moral issue such as sleep deprivation, giving birth, or parenting can trigger schizophrenic symptoms.[43]

Although those with schizophrenia do sin, as a group they have not sinned any more than other people.[44] More often they are the victims of living in a sinful society made up of sinful individuals. They are always fragile people in a rough and stressful world deserving our love, understanding and support.

Conclusions

The best medical position on schizophrenia is that it involves a genetic predisposition or weakness coupled with a stress factor that pushes a person over a threshold into schizophrenic symptoms. Acceptance of this view could help pastors and lay people minister to families of consumers.

Christians have to understand a problem correctly in order to apply the Bible to it. If they do not, there can be a misapplication that causes great harm. Biblical evidence allows a view that schizophrenia is largely a medical problem. In general, ministry to the families of people with schizophrenia can adopt models patterned after ministry to families faced with other chronic medical problems. Although stress from wrong activities could possibly be a factor that triggers schizophrenia, stress equally arises from being the victim of wrongdoing or from non-moral pressures in life. Having schizophrenia in and of itself is not a matter of sin. Schizophrenia is best classed under the theological category of a human infirmity or limitation. Christians with schizophrenia experience great spiritual struggles and can also win great spiritual victories. Their families also have great struggles. We will consider the family's emotional response to schizophrenia in the next chapter.

---

[43]Ibid.

[44]Welch and I would disagree on some secondary theological points and conclusions about schizophrenia, but he agrees that those with mental problems do not have greater sins than the rest of the human race for we all have a wicked side. Welch, *Counselor's Guide*, 235.

Questions and Thoughts to Consider from Chapter Two

Until recently psychologists/psychiatrists cast blame upon families for causing mental illnesses. Is it possible that their conclusions influenced the clergy so that some of the ignorance in the church could be traced back to a shared ignorance on the part of all in past decades?

What do you think of the classification of schizophrenia as an infirmity rather than a sin?

Do you believe those with schizophrenia are capable of great spiritual battles and also great victories?

Assuming you accept the Bible's authority, how would you handle the truth "all have sinned" as it applies to those with schizophrenia?

Newer medicines have not cured schizophrenia, but they have improved the lives of those who have it. How can Christians minister to consumers?

Chapter Three

Emotional Responses In the Family

Schizophrenia torments a family. Those who have never faced the curse of this brain disorder cannot fully understand the pain.

"God must have been having a bad day," a father recently wrote me, "when He allowed schizophrenia to come into existence." It is a sentiment shared by most mothers and fathers who have faced the specter of this disease. An ordeal of greater magnitude than most people ever must face, schizophrenia challenges not only parents' equilibrium, economics, and ingenuity, as do many chronic illnesses, but their psychological and theological core as well. Schizophrenia, it may be said, is a job for Job.[45]

In 1982 Abigail Van Buren, author of "Dear Abby," asked families to share their experiences concerning living with a mentally ill relative. The responses display deepness of pain. Dear Abby concludes:

The immense grief of these families over lost dreams and hopes for a promising child or beloved spouse and the suffering caused by a mentally ill parent or sibling are cruelly aggravated by undeserved guilt and shame, by alienation from friends and neighbors, by severe financial drain, and by the paucity of desperately needed resources. Many respondents said that they did not receive the support they needed from either the helping professions or from psychiatric and social institutions.

The message is loud and clear: The family of the chronically mentally ill person cannot carry such responsibility alone.[46]

---

[45]Walsh, *Schizophrenia*, 9. This quote is from the introduction by E. Fuller Torrey.

[46]*A Family Affair: Helping Families Cope with Mental Illness,* (New York: Brunner/Mazel, 1986), xii-xiii.

Emotional responses to the schizophrenia of a loved one parallel bereavement. I know this both from personal experience and research. My two sons remind me of the past and the relationship I had with my brother. I often want the "old" Mark back, but that Mark is gone. I also feel cheated because I will never be an uncle to his children. Families commonly explain they feel as if a loved one is dying. "It is as though he had a terminal illness, except he never dies."[47] Experts tell a family what to expect.

> Of course, with a chronically mentally ill relative the mourning process is never completed; rather, periods of relative quiet and acceptance are interspersed with episodes of renewed grief stimulated, perhaps, by the accomplishment of a peer, or a birthday, or some other seemingly innocuous event.[48]

Despite the fact that many Christians have no firsthand experience with mental illness, all can identify with the emotions associated with death. All should be able to agree that the Scriptures give comfort for those with such emotions.

Sometimes families feel guilt over the death of a loved one. They wonder if they could have done more to keep their relative alive. Families of those with schizophrenia might also agonize over guilt.

Guilt/Shame

Legitimate guilt is to the soul what pain is to the body. Guilt alerts us that something is wrong. When the Bible commands or prohibits a certain action or attitude, failure to comply leads to true guilt. The solution to true guilt is faith in Jesus Christ, God the Son, who paid for our sins on the cross and arose from the dead. He took all punishment for our guilt so that we can be forgiven and free of guilt.

However, false guilt occurs when we feel guilty for not measuring up to a purely man-made standard (e.g. legalism induces false guilt) or

---

[47]Walsh, *Schizophrenia,* 34.

[48]Bernheim, *Working with Families of the Mentally Ill,* 19-20.

even to self-imposed false standards that do not actually come from the Bible. People can also feel guilty when they have been victimized. Rape victims commonly undergo false guilt. Children of divorce often accept guilt for the home's demise. The decision to move grandmother into a nursing home causes false guilt. One who injures or kills another in a car accident may feel false guilt even though his actions were unintentional. Christian families of people with schizophrenia suffer from tremendous feelings of guilt. They may have had to call the police to secure a loved one. Commitment laws are such that our family ended up prosecuting my brother so he could enter a hospital. The need to drug and/or institutionalize a relative causes guilt. Families experience a vague sense of guilt wondering whether they could do more (or spend more) to find a cure. They may feel guilt for feeling embarrassed over their relative. Perhaps the most common guilt feelings arise over concern that the family caused mental illness. For a long time I felt guilty for being an achiever. I wondered if Mark got sick because of the stress involved in trying to attain my accomplishments. Above all else, families must look to the Bible for authentic standards of right and wrong. We may feel guilt over a situation or action, but unless the Scripture labels it as sin, we have not sinned. Admitting a family member for psychiatric care is morally indistinct from admitting a family member for a gall bladder operation. Taking drugs to control hallucinations is as morally neutral as taking drugs for asthma. Those who feel guilt over using medical professionals for psychiatric care might want to read *Can We Trust Psychology?* by Gary Collins to get a balanced view of the value of medical care for mental illness.[49]

Concern over family causation of schizophrenia generates the greatest amount of guilt. Most experts conclude biological problems are the main factor in mental illness. A minority disagree.[50] However, evidence points to a genetic predisposition as the primary cause for schizophrenia, and new technology will probably make the case for a strong biological factor in causation more firm each year (see Chapter 2).

---

[49]Collins neither worships secular therapy as a new religion nor rejects all its insights.

[50]Virtually all of the sources listed in the bibliography argue for a strong medical cause. The exceptions are David Oppenheimer, who accepts a family causation view, and Edward T. Welch, who argues for schizophrenia beginning as a spiritual/emotional problem that also becomes a medical problem.

My personal opinion is that the debate over the causes of schizophrenia parallels the debate over linking smoking to cancer. Initial studies were met with stiff objections by those with a vested interest in the issue. However, medical evidence accumulated over decades will probably make those who blame families for schizophrenia look as absurd as those who still defend tobacco. Some psychoanalysts have built careers on blaming mom. They are not likely to surrender easily. Although we definitely need more research, those who argue for family causation of schizophrenia have at best an uphill struggle. More probably, they fight for a hopeless position.

Those in Christian circles could also have a problem but may not realize it. I believe that many ministers gravitate toward the family causation position because they want to maintain human responsibility and accountability for behavior. Their motives and goals are good, but one can reject family causation of mental illness and still view those involved with a schizophrenic disorder morally accountable as I have tried to do in Chapter Two, pp. 39-42. It is too easy for Christians to see schizophrenia as a symptom of the decline in the family. Mental illness is assumed to arise only in dysfunctional families. However, in cases of Christian families with loved ones who have schizophrenia, a family causation theory is tantamount to concluding that a Christian upbringing causes mental illness. My parents prayed and had family devotions. They took us to Sunday School, Vacation Bible School and summer camp. We had unconditional love, plenty of family recreation, and an absence of family conflict. How would a theory that rests totally on family causation explain one son's residence in a mental hospital while another son takes a seminary degree as class valedictorian? Lionel Aldridge had played professional football for the Green Bay Packers and worked as a news broadcaster. Then he suffered schizophrenia. In cases where a person achieves and then has schizophrenia, shall we credit parents for the years of progress and then fault them for a disorder which their child develops in adulthood?[51]

Some may feel blaming families bolsters the legitimate principle of human responsibility and accountability. However, the family

---

[51]"News from Medicine: Peace of Mind" gives Mr. Adlridge's moving story. He found help for his illness through both medical and Biblical therapy.

causation view also ends up with the uncomfortable position that Christian child-rearing can cause mental illness. Theologically, there need not be any preference for either family causation or biological causation. Scientific evidence indicates that schizophrenia stems from a brain disorder.

Those who blame schizophrenia on families may neither do so with any great arsenal of scientific facts nor claim theological support. A dogmatic and stern denunciation of families would be impossible to justify from Scripture or from scientific evidence. Condemnation, meanness and cruelty towards suffering people on prejudice alone is a real moral issue.[52] Mental retardation, Alzheimer's or schizophrenia are not primarily moral issues, but instead they are medical ones.

If you feel guilt over a relative's schizophrenia, remember that the Bible alone defines sin. We must realize that we can feel guilt without an objective basis for guilt. It may even be true that your family had severe spiritual defects, but a brain disorder was probably not one of its adverse affects. At the most, such failures triggered a response because of a pre-existing genetic weakness. Stress from a non-moral source, such as pressures in college or a broken engagement, would perhaps have also brought on the same disorder. You may have sinned against God or your relative. There is a need to obtain forgiveness from God by confessing those sins. Yet, God does not want us to suffer the needless pain of false guilt that can emanate from tragedies that we did not directly or intentionally cause or for sins that have already been confessed and forgiven. He wants us to enjoy His grace and unconditional love.

- For if our hearts condemn us, God is greater than our heart, and knoweth all things. (1 John 3:20 KJV).

---

[52]Even if one wishes to accept the view that schizophrenia's origin is primarily a matter of personal or family weaknesses/sins, there still must be caution against a wholesale condemnation of those with schizophrenia and their families. Even if such views could not be absolutely disproved, they cannot be proven with any great certainty either! In practice there is no justification whatsoever to approach consumers or their families with condemnation. Regardless of debate as to its origin, these people need Christian compassion and not additional pain.

Anger

Close relatives of those with schizophrenia experience anger. They might be angry at the consumer for his irritable behavior, angry at other family members who refuse to share in the burdens of caregiving, angry at doctors or the mental health system, angry at the illness, angry over increased cost and work, angry at feeling trapped, and even angry at God or His representatives— the church or its minister. The Bible distinguishes between righteous anger and sinful anger. Those who are close to one with schizophrenic symptoms may feel both.

Obviously, God's own anger proves the concept of righteous anger (Ex. 4:14; Mark 3:5; Rom. 1:18). Righteous anger arises when God's standards of justice and holiness have been violated as opposed to "self" being offended. Paul commands us to "abhor evil" (Rom. 12:9; see also Ps. 97:10a, 139:20-24 and Amos 5:15a). Righteous anger is also long suffering and compassionate. God's anger comes after initial patience. God punished Israel for rejecting her Savior but only after extreme longsuffering on His part.

- O Jerusalem, Jerusalem, who kills the prophets and stones those who are sent to her! How often I wanted to gather your children together, the way a hen gathers her chicks under her wings, and you were unwilling. Behold, your house is being left to you desolate (Matthew 23:37-38)

Aspects of schizophrenia call for righteous anger. Families soon discover plenty of injustices and incompetencies in the mental health care system. Some "professionals" are truly disgusting. Maryellen Walsh tells of unnecessary pain heaped upon families.

Social workers told us we caused it.

The hospital told us we couldn't visit for three months. It was clear they thought we would contaminate him.

I can't answer your questions about mental health professionals, it is too hard...thinking of how they treated us.[53]

Rev. John Cannon, past president of the Georgia Alliance for the Mentally Ill, gives a detailed and personal account.

In the early days of my son's illness, the commonly accepted theories of the cause of mental illness emphasized environmental factors such as "poor parenting" or perhaps "emotional or physical abuse." We heard about the "Schizophrenigenic mother" and the "ineffectual father" and later "pathological families," "identified patients," and "double binds." These only increased our guilt, sent us examining ourselves for failures and too often blaming each other. One of the most devastating experiences I have ever experienced was the night a counselor placed two chairs in the middle of her office, instructed me to sit in one and my son in the other and said, "Now, apologize to your son for what you have done to him." Unfortunately, in spite of recent research, these theories still are widely held. Recently, I was leading an inservice training session at a community mental health center. One staff member stated categorically, "Families are usually sicker than the patients." Such attitudes by some mental health professionals have added to the burden of guilt and failure experienced by families.[54]

In addition to anger over wrongs, families may feel a general anger over the very existence of brain disorders. The Greek text of John 11:33 indicates the Lord Jesus was disturbed by the disease and death of his friend, Lazarus. When he saw relatives weeping over Lazarus, "He was deeply moved in spirit and was troubled." The word "troubled" can mean "indignant." Jesus felt indignant at what sin has wrought in human life. He was mad over the very existence of sickness.

---

[53]Walsh, *Schizophrenia*, 36.

[54]Rev. John M. Cannon, "Pastoral Care for the Families of the Mentally Ill," *The Journal of Pastoral Care*, XLIV, no. 3 (Fall 1990): 215-216.

Some aspects of mental illness arouse righteous anger. It is normal to be upset over diseases or mistreatment by others. However, the handling of righteous anger is tricky. We can respond to a wrong with a sin of our own. The Bible might allow righteous anger, but it never allows bitterness (Eph. 4:31; Heb. 12:15). Paul allows for a right kind of anger but not for the sin of a lasting grudge.

- Be angry, and yet do not let the sun go down on your anger (Eph. 4:26).

If your anger turns into the paralysis of bitterness, you have suffered for nothing. Righteous anger creates a strong motivation for doing good. If you are angry over the presence of schizophrenia or some mistreatment received from the public or professionals or even church members, you can best handle that anger by turning it into energy for ministry to consumers and their families. This may take the form of helping a particular family or joining a support or advocacy group. If anger creates a burden and motivation to work, then we benefit from anger. If we end up in bitterness seeking revenge rather than change, our initial righteous anger has become sinful anger. It helps no one.

Anger also brings many opportunities for rationalization. Often we evaluate our anger as righteous when it is really sinful. We are neither objecting to a violation of God's holy standards, nor have we begun with initial longsuffering. We are just sinfully angry and try to justify it with a claim to righteous anger. Consider whether your anger arose over genuine sins inflicted against you or over frustration with non-sinful human limitations. As much as possible, we have to be objective, fair, and possess realistic expectations. Maybe the afflicted loved one cannot control his irritating behavior. Maybe mental health professionals are really giving their best efforts but have limited abilities to help. Maybe friends are not actually unsympathetic and cruel; rather, they just feel awkward and do not know how to help. The golden rule may apply. Would you feel anger was righteous if you had been in the role of the person who made you angry? Put yourself into the role of the doctor, consumer, social worker, family, or church member. Would you have done any better? Anger with people who have done nothing wrong is quite unjustified and will need to be confessed to God and perhaps to people offended by the anger. It is hard to believe that an explanation of the stresses associated with dealing with a relative's mental illness plus an appeal for forgiveness would not meet with a warm response. In the rare cases where it does not, the burden of sin must rest on the unforgiving party. Prayer for that person is the primary avenue left in normalizing the strained relationship. The best outcome to an incident of sinful anger is forgiveness and renewed harmony in relationships. This is also true when our anger focuses on God.

Christian families who have a relative suffering from schizophrenia may experience anger at God for permitting brain disorders in a fallen world. Even secular books note anger with God as a common reaction to mental illness in the family.

People with a religious faith may question how God could allow this to happen to them. They may feel that it is a terrible sin to be angry with God or they may fear that they have lost their faith. Such feelings may deprive them of the strength and reassurance faith offers at just the time when they need it most. To struggle with such questions is part of the experience of faith.

Said a minister, "I wonder how God could do this to me. I haven't been perfect, but I've done the best I could. And I love my wife. But then I think I have no right to question God. For me that is the hardest part. I think I must be a very weak person to question God."[55]

Family members search for an explanation of the illness outside of their own behavior as well, and are often plagued with feelings of anger--at the ill relative who is often seen as malingering or manipulative, at other family members, at the ineffective professional "helpers," at unsupportive extended family or friends, at God. Typically, anger and guilt go hand in hand, as one leads to the other in a painful, debilitating cycle.[56]

---

[55]Mace, *The 36 Hour Day,* 229.

[56]Bernheim, *Working with Families of the Mentally Ill,* 19.

Consider the perplexity and anguish expressed in this quote recorded by social worker Julie Tallard Johnson: "I get to the part in 'The Lord's Prayer' that says, 'Thy will be done,' and I think 'No! Not if *this* is His will.' *Why* I ask, does God permit such a horrible thing to happen to someone?"[57]

Although anger with God cannot be approved, it must be accepted as reality. Denial or repression of anger against God is not helpful towards a solution. The Bible gives many expressions of feelings that God has been unfair.

> • Have I sinned? What have I done to Thee, O watcher of men? Why hast Thou set me as Thy target, so that I am a burden to myself (Job 7:20)?

> • According to Thy knowledge I am indeed not guilty; Yet there is no deliverance from Thy hand (Job 10:7).

> • Know then that God has wronged me, and has closed His net around me (Job 19:6).

> • How long, O LORD? Wilt Thou forget me forever? How long wilt Thou hide Thy face from me? (Psa. 13:1)

> • Why do you say, O Jacob, and assert, O Israel, "My way is hidden from the LORD, and the justice due me escapes the notice of my God"? (Isa. 40:27).

> • O LORD, Thou hast deceived me and I was deceived; Thou hast overcome me and prevailed. I have become a laughingstock all day long; everyone mocks me (Jer. 20:7).

If we find ourselves angry with God, we are better off admitting rather than denying the feelings. We may have deep intellectual convictions about God's righteousness but still feel upset because He allows schizophrenia. The very recognition that fact and feelings are

---

[57]Julie Tallard Johnson, *Hidden Victims* (New York: Doubleday, 1988), 78.

separate may help. Feeling God has been unfair does not mean that He is actually unfair.

We also know the Bible gives many reasons why God might allow His children to suffer (see Chapter Four). Although a family may not be emotionally able to receive these truths during the initial period of a relative's mental illness, eventually there may be some understanding of God's purposes for allowing hardship. Just knowing that God has good purposes for suffering should help alleviate anger towards Him.

Furthermore, the doctrine of God's sovereignty includes the idea that God knows all things potential, as well as things actual. Not only does He know the future, God also knows all potential futures that would have occurred had history been different (see 1 Sam. 23:11-12; 2 Sam. 12:8; Psa. 81:13-15; Jer. 1:5, 38:17-20; Ezek. 3:5-7; Matt. 11:21-24). If Jesus had preached in Tyre and Sidon, they would have repented. Most of these examples concern the future destruction of nations. God also knows the potential future for individuals. Matthew 11:21-24 concerns the behavior of individuals. He knows what might have been.

God knows what might have been if a person or family never experienced mental illness. We really do not. We assume life would have been better. God knows.

The story is told of a pastor visiting a sick newborn and mother in the hospital. He prayed that the baby live "If it is within God's will." The mother angrily denied any concern for God's will. The baby survived. He grew. He became a mass murderer. While God's purposes in this story are still ultimately hidden, we can see in theory how humans may not know what is best. God's way is superior even if it involves hardship. Sometimes a Christian must just trust Him.

As a good father, God allows us to ask freely, but wisdom demands that any divine veto of our prayers will find our acceptance. We as ignorant children can ask for an outcome that is not really in our best interest. It may be fine to ask, but ask with the attitude that the heavenly Father knows best even if He has permitted schizophrenia. Our feelings of anger over God's supposed unfairness do not make Him unfair. He has taught us about good outcomes to suffering, and He knows all potential futures. In heaven Christian relatives of those with schizophrenia will learn how God's permission to allow a brain disorder was the best course of all potential outcomes.

- Oh, the depth of the riches both of the wisdom and knowledge of God! How unsearchable are His judgments and unfathomable His ways (Rom. 11:33)!

God's righteousness is equaled only by His grace. When believers are angry at Him, He will forgive when we confess (1 John 1:9). You may need to confess anger toward God. Remember, He forgives completely. It is not right to presume upon God's grace, but when we need to lean on His grace, He invites us to lean hard. Accept His forgiveness. Then enjoy His forgiveness. Get over the sinful anger. Then go on in your spiritual life. After confession of sinful anger, reject any future guilt for even being angry at God. He understands, forgives, and loves us anyway.

Loneliness

Families of a person with mental illness often suffer in silent isolation. Sometimes they struggle with embarrassment over their relative. In turn, friends feel awkward. They do not know what to say or how to help, so they frequently withdraw. The resulting social situation parallels ancient attitudes toward leprosy.

The burden of caregiving reinforces withdrawal from social contact. The family might fear leaving a consumer at home alone. They are trapped.

I believe that our church felt we had spiritual problems because of decreased church attendance. Absence from services seemed to be another symptom of an unspiritual home. Perhaps the same problem that brought on the mental illness? In reality, care for a person with schizophrenia can become so demanding that the family essentially adopts the role of a "shut-in." Churches understand how old age gives a person an excuse for withdrawal from attendance. Would anyone leave a young adult home alone if he had once tried to set fire to the home or castrate himself? Withdrawal is harmful, but the tendency can actually be a sign of family devotion coupled with the stigma and confusion of mental illness in a home.

A minister or church family need not have expertise on schizophrenia to help families who struggle with it.[58] Christians should not automatically conclude suffering families want to be left alone. Their shyness is more probably the result of shame, stigma, and deep involvement in care for their relatives. Families will naturally have a tendency to withdraw. When the church responds with avoidance of its own, the end is a double tragedy in that fellowship is also severed at a time the family needs much support. Even if a minister or church does not have all the answers, inadequacy should not increase avoidance. Listening itself is a ministry. Weeping with those who weep is a ministry. Reminding the suffering of simple Bible truths is a ministry. Learning how to supervise a person with severe schizophrenia would be a valuable ministry as families need some respite to avoid burnout.

- Rejoice with those who rejoice, and weep with those who weep (Rom. 12:15).

- Bear one another's burdens, and thus fulfill the law of Christ (Gal.6:2).

- ... not forsaking our own assembling together, as is the habit of some, but encouraging one another; and all the more, as you see the day drawing near (Heb. 10:25).

If you find yourself lonely, do not let false shame prevent you from looking to others for support. Most cities have chapters of the Alliance for the Mentally Ill. Most churches will respond in friendship and love once enlightened about the facts of schizophrenia. If people are

---

[58]"With our strong tendency to professionalize all human problems, we lose sight of the part played by an array of informal caregivers; family members, friends, neighbors, clergy, co-workers..." Agnes B. Hat-field, "Social Support and Family Coping," *Families of the Mentally Ill*, 193; see also *The Journal of Pastoral Care*, XLIV, no.2 (Summer, 1990), 158-159 for excellent comments about the need for care from non-medical friends.

reserved, try to understand that many people would like to show concern but feel awkward. Maybe you can educate them and in the process form deeper friendships.

Stress

"Stress constituted the most common emotional response in the family," says one authority on mental illness[59]. Couples must be warned of a tendency for family conflicts over a child's schizophrenia to end in divorce. While my parents love each other and have had a stable marriage for nearly 40 years, Mark's mental illness caused disagreements. Who or what caused the condition? Should he live at home, in an institution, or in his own place? Have we been too lenient or too hard on him? I noticed that my parents would often switch their viewpoint and contend for a position they rejected only a few months earlier. Families need preparation for and resistance to the tendency for schizophrenia to increase tension in the home. Pressures always increase, and 20% of families report that the stress was a "threat to parents' marriage."[60]

> The strain of the demands and behavior of the ill person may cause healthy family members to drift apart, to fight with one another over the ill member, and to generally become more isolated. The splitting up of the family into individuals struggling with one another further increases the burdens of chronic care. Sometimes the tension and divisiveness become so great that family members may separate and divorce.[61]

> The presence of a mentally ill member tends to both provoke conflict between other family members and magnify the normal conflicts that occur in any case.[62]

---

[59]Bernheim, *Working With Families of the Mentally Ill*, 10.

[60]Ibid., 8.

[61]Bernheim, *The Caring Family*, 73.

[62]Bernheim, *Working with Families of the Mentally Ill*, 22.

Maintaining a good marriage is often not easy, and caring for a person with a dementing illness can make it much more difficult. It may mean more financial burdens and less time to talk, to go out, and to make love. It may entail being involved with your in-laws, having more things to disagree over, often being tired, and short-changing the children. It can mean having to include a difficult, disagreeable, seemingly demanding, and sick person in your lives.[63]

Married couples can expect increased occasions for conflict over decisions about care. It helps if both will work at attacking problems not personalities. In reality both husband and wife probably have the best intentions. If you disagree with your spouse on a course of action, at least appreciate a situation where he or she has pure motives and really loves the family.

Ministers have weaknesses in specific counseling for families in a crisis over a schizophrenic illness. However, ministers are often experts on marriage counseling. If your minister accepts the Bible as the Word of God, you would be wise to get some counseling on Biblical communication, decision-making, and the roles of husband/wife.[64] Ask for help before any more conflicts arise. If you have a person with severe schizophrenia in your family, the conflicts will come.

Marital conflict is not the only problem stress over schizophrenia brings. You could also work until you literally collapse. The demands of caring for one with a mental illness can cause physical illness. Relatives of a person with schizophrenia indeed have heavy responsibilities. Yet, you need to realize your limitations. All of us have limitations in wisdom and strength. Dedication to care is admirable and helpful. Yet, extreme sacrifice for a loved one is not going to cure a brain disorder, but burnout on your part will diminish the quality of care you can give.Get enough rest. One of the dilemmas families often face is that the care giver may not get enough rest or may

---

[63]Mace, *The 36 Hour Day*, 214. Her comments about Alzheimer's disease seem to apply to family situations involving schizophrenia.

[64]The author has Bible study notes for all of these topics. Write Westcliff Bible Church, P.O. Box 1521, Amarillo, TX, 79105.

not have the opportunity to get away from his care giving responsibilities. This can make the caregiver less patient and less able to tolerate irritating behaviors. If things are getting out of hand, ask yourself if this is happening to you. If so, you may want to focus on finding ways to get more rest or more frequent breaks from your care giving responsibilities. We recognize that this is difficult to arrange.[65]

Balance makes life manageable. Yes, we must help our relatives. But God alone can part the Red Sea. Acceptance of our limitations and realistic expectations will prevent additional casualties. You will need respite from caregiving labors. You will need rest. You will need exercise. Husbands and wives need time alone. You have my permission and blessing to pester your church for some volunteers to supervise while you get a break. You need the time off. The church needs the ministry experience.

Fear

Schizophrenia fosters great fears. Family members may or may not fear their relative, but they always fear the future. Will he or she kill himself? What happens if there is a refusal to take medication? Will medicine cause harmful side affects? How will a son or daughter fare should the parents die? Will a younger child also develop schizophrenia? If the ill person wanders off, will he join the ranks of street people? Will we ever see him/her again? How will we pay for treatment? Some of these questions have partial answers. One out of ten with schizophrenia commits suicide.[66] Approximately 30-40% of the homeless suffer mental illness.[67] The chart in Chapter Two, page 24 lists the probabilities of other family members getting schizophrenia.

Cold statistical answers do little toward alleviating a family's fears. Scriptures give much more hope than statistical analysis. Fears that arise among Christian families of people who have schizophrenia have the same solution as fears from any other source. Fear stops when faith

---

[65]Mace, *The 36 Hour Day*, 33.

[66]Torrey, *Surviving Schizophrenia*, 117; and Isaac, *Madness in the Streets*, 281.

[67]Isaac, *Madness in the Streets*, 4-5.

increases. Fear also evaporates when the person has deep assurance of God's love.

•Let not your heart be troubled; believe in God, believe also in Me .... Peace I leave with you; My peace I give to you; not as the world gives, do I give to you. Let not your heart be troubled, nor let it be fearful (John 14:1,27).

• Be anxious for nothing, but in everything by prayer and supplication with thanksgiving let your requests be made known to God. And the peace of God, which surpasses all comprehension, shall guard your heart and your minds in Christ Jesus. Finally, brethren, whatever is true, whatever is honorable, whatever is right, whatever is pure, whatever is lovely, whatever is of good repute, if there is any excellence and if anything worthy of praise, let your mind dwell on these things. The things you have learned and received and heard and seen in me, practice these things; and the God of peace shall be with you (Phil. 4:6-9).

• There is no fear in love; but perfect love casts out fear... (1 John. 4:18).

• Cast your burden upon the LORD, and He will sustain you; He will never allow the righteous to be shaken (Psa. 55:22).

• ... casting all our anxiety upon Him, because He cares for you (1 Peter 5:7).

Faith is only as good as its object. If I trust an airplane to take me to Chicago, my faith is valid if I am in a quality aircraft with an expert pilot. Jesus Christ is the object of Christian faith. He has proven Himself wise, ethical, and completely trustworthy. We can trust in His promise to save those who accept Him as Savior. We can trust His unconditional love for believers. If we have deep confidence that God really loves us, we will experience less fear. If we have faith in Him to take care of matters beyond our control, we will have less fear.

Troubles, such as having schizophrenia in a family, force Christians to consider what they really think of Jesus Christ. If we still find Him dependable, we will be able to manage any fear.

Matthew 6:34 gives us the wise principle of tackling each days problems and refusing to endure terror over what might happen in the future. Most fear involves what could, but what may never, happen. A better approach is to concentrate on a present problem and leave an unknown future to God.

> • Therefore do not be anxious for tomorrow; for tomorrow will care for itself. Each day has enough trouble of its own (Matt. 6:34).

Depression

Of course, dangers of depression stalk the families involved with a schizophrenic illness. I do not refer to a medically based depression. I mean depression caused by life's hardships. All of the preceding emotional reactions tend to bring on depression. Let me repeat the outline of a lecture I gave at St. Anthony's Hospital in Amarillo, Texas, "Biblical Causes of Depression." You will see why we are studying depression at this point.

1. **Guilt** - Both true guilt and false guilt bring on depression. The guilt in King David after his adultery with Bathsheba drove him into depression.

> • For my iniquities are gone over my head; as a heavy burden they weigh too much for me.... I am bent over and greatly bowed down; I go mourning all day long.... I am benumbed and badly crushed; I groan because of the agitation of my heart (Psa. 38:4,6 and 8).

> • Restore to me the joy of Thy salvation, and sustain me with a willing spirit (Psa. 51:12).

David did not lose his salvation because of guilt, but he lost the joy of his salvation. The solution for true guilt is faith in the Lord Jesus

Christ and His death on the cross to pay for our sins. Those who are already believers must also confess their sins to God the Father (1 John 1:9). If we comply with these teachings, God promises total forgiveness with no more need to feel any true guilt.

False guilt also brings feelings of condemnation with resulting depression (1 Jn. 3:20). The solution, as has been explained above, lies in making the Bible alone our standard of morality (see pp.49-53). If we have committed no sin, the guilt is false. Much of the guilt among families of those with schizophrenia is needless; therefore, depression is also needless.

2. **Anger** - The story of Jonah shows that anger and resentment lead to depression. In Jonah 4:1-3, Jonah seethes in anger over God's mercy towards the hated Assyrians. He is so mad he wants to die!

• But it greatly displeased Jonah, and he became angry. And he prayed to the LORD and said, "Please LORD, was not this what I said while I was still in my own country? Therefore, in order to forestall this I fled to Tarshish, for I know that Thou are a gracious and compassionate God, slow to anger and abundant in lovingkindness, and one who relents concerning calamity. Therefore now, O LORD, please take my life from me, for death is better to me than life" (Jonah 4:1-3).

Anger can cause serious depression. Christians must direct righteous anger into motivation for change. Sinful anger should be admitted and confessed to obtain God's complete forgiveness. If we fail to handle anger Biblically, we could end up as depressed as Jonah.

3. **Loneliness** - The Prophet Elijah's depression also caused him to wish for death. Loneliness was a primary factor in his serious depression.

• But he himself went a day's journey into the wilderness, and came and sat down under a juniper tree; and he requested for himself that he might die, and said, "It is enough; now, O Lord, take my life, for I am not better than my fathers..." Then he came there to a cave, and lodged there; and behold, the word of the LORD came to him, and He said to him, "What are you doing here, Elijah?" And he said, "I have been very zealous for the LORD, the God of hosts; for the sons of Israel have forsaken Thy covenant, torn down Thine altars and killed Thy prophets with the sword. And I alone am left; and they seek my life, to take it away" (1 Kings 19:4,9 and 10).

Loneliness can twist our personalities. Refuse to allow schizophrenia to push you into isolation. Others do care. You can find them at church or at family support groups. The desire to reach out to people with your pain will help save you from depression.

4. **Stress** - Stress from perfectionism also generates depression. The Bible shows this in Numbers 11. Moses believed the whole world rested on his shoulders. The truth is that he could not handle such massive burdens. God gave him great responsibility, but God never asked him to do the impossible. Moses just took that burden upon himself. Modern perfectionists make the same mistake and suffer depression for it.

- So Moses said to the LORD, "Why hast Thou been so hard on Thy servant? And why have I not found favor in Thy sight, that Thou hast laid the burden of all this people on me? Was it I who conceived all this people? Was it I who brought them forth, that Thou shouldest say to me, 'Carry them in your bosom as a nurse carries a nursing infant, to the land which Thou didst swear to their fathers'? "Where am I to get meat to give to all this people? For they weep before me, saying, 'Give us meat that we may eat!' "I alone am not able to carry all this people, because it is too burdensome for me. So if Thou art going to deal thus with me, please kill me at once, if I have found favor in Thy sight, and do not let me see my wretchedness" (Numbers 11:11-15).

Perfectionism will drive relatives of a person with schizophrenia into deep depression. God does not call upon his children to do the impossible, but we can place that burden on ourselves. We must do our best to care for our loved ones. Yet, if we think extra sacrifice will achieve the impossible, we end up depressed.

Perfectionism will drive relatives of a person with schizophrenia into deep depression. God does not call upon his children to do the impossible, but we can place that burden on ourselves. We must do our best to care for our loved ones. Yet, if we think extra sacrifice will achieve the impossible, we end up depressed.

Maybe God did not call you to cure schizophrenia. Realistic expectations and goals reduce depression.

- Why are you downcast, O my soul? Why so disturbed within me? Put your hope in God, for I will yet praise him, my Savior and my God (Psa. 42:5 NIV).

Faith in Christ is of extreme importance both for eternal salvation and emotional well being. Those who have deep confidence in God will be able to handle fear and avoid another cause for depression. Those who refuse faith in Christ just add to their fears and make escape from depression impossible.

Our handling of the first five emotions discussed in this section (guilt, anger, loneliness, stress, and fear) determine susceptibility to depression. Schizophrenia creates great problems for families and friends. Our emotional struggles cannot be made easy. Nevertheless, God's Word teaches the best way to handle our emotions. Acceptance of Biblical wisdom makes a tough situation easier. Indifference to this wisdom makes it hopeless.

Two more emotional responses remain: denial and confusion. The Bible deals less directly with them, but reason alone gives us some answers.

Denial

No one wants to accept the fact that a loved one has schizophrenia. Some hope against hope that it is not true. Yet, after a duration of symptoms, after the second opinion has been rendered, families must accept the truth. How can there be resolve to help the loved one or ability to cope with our emotions if we deny the reality of illness?

Sometimes we must not only accept the illness but also accept realistic expectations for a cure. New generations of medicine continue to improve the outcome for schizophrenia, but the disorder still produces limitations. Acceptance of reality produces the assurance that a family is doing its best. Realistic expectations of a consumer's abilities improve a family's level of toleration for what otherwise would be irritating behavior.

The serenity prayer gives a wise course to follow with any chronic disorder. "God grant me the serenity to accept the things I cannot change, the courage to change the things I can, and the wisdom to know the difference."

Confusion

My brother's mental illness created great confusion in our household. We wrestled with spiritual questions, medical questions, practical questions (such as the best housing for Mark and how to communicate with a person who hears voices), financial questions and even legal questions.

If you have just received a diagnosis of schizophrenia in your family, you are probably experiencing the same confusion. Perhaps the advice given by various family members is conflicting and your confusion is only intensified. Our relatives told us more hard work on the farm, or vitamins, or counseling might fix schizophrenia.

While all your questions may not have answers, there is more wisdom about schizophrenia than there was a few decades ago. Some of the confusion will disappear with a few hours spent on reading material listed in the bibliography. Deeper understanding would arise from attendance at local Alliance for the Mentally Ill meetings. Some aspects of mental illness remain mysterious, but no one need endure the darkest of confusion. Many fellow families who have had misfortune with schizophrenia are capable of giving wise counsel and most eager to reduce the confusion of others by sharing their insight. In Chapter Four, I will share some of my insight into the perplexing question of why God allows His people to suffer.

Questions and Thoughts to consider from Chapter Three

1. Do you believe a family's experience with schizophrenia can be similar to the grieving process after a death?

2. Does your concept of God include the belief that He desires to forgive?

3. Can you think of specific examples of false guilt arising from your family's experience with schizophrenia?

4. Have you experienced anger at God over the hardships in your family? Can you acknowledge this anger without necessarily approving it?

5. Do you think it is true that friends who have no professional training in mental health care can still be helpful to families of those with schizophrenia?

6. Has your relative's schizophrenia put a strain on your marriage?

Chapter Four

"My God, My God, Why...?"

Serious mental illnesses affect one in four American families.[68] Two million people suffer from schizophrenia.[69] Christian ministry must not ignore them or classify them as having a sort of modern leprosy. Christian ministry and pastoral care certainly should extend to the families of any chronically struggling person. Indeed, one almost has to try to avoid such families. Consider that "25 percent of all beds in our hospitals are filled by mentally ill patients—more than beds for the victims of heart disease, cancer, and respiratory ailments combined."[70]

These families deserve care from church members and pastors. Fortunately, Scripture addresses their most common emotional needs. The Word of God has answers when psychology alone has reached its limitations. A totally secular approach cannot begin to answer the problem of pain. From an atheist's or agnostic's perspective, suffering is dumb, capricious, nonsense. Christianity has better answers as to why bad things happen to good people.

Every family of a person with schizophrenia will ask the question, "Why?" Believers may feel guilt for even having such thoughts. Yet, when asked from a spirit of inquiry as opposed to one of hostility, the question, "Why have you forsaken me?", has validity. King David of the Old Testament and the Lord Jesus Christ of the New Testament prove the question is legitimate (see Psa. 22:1; Matt. 27:46).

---

[68]"Texas Alliance for the Mentally Ill," (Austin, TX: TEXAMI, n.d.).

[69]Walsh, *Schizophrenia*, 52.

[70]"Texas Alliance for the Mentally Ill," see also: Rael Jean Isaac and Virginia C. Armat, *Madness in the Streets*, (New York: The Free Press, a division of MacMillian, 1990) 9. "...a recent CBS-New York Times poll found that only 1% of respondents thought mental illness was a major health problem! This despite the fact that even now, in the era of radical deinstitutionalization, schizophrenia still accounts for 40% of *all* long-term hospital beds."

Ancient people believed that punishment from a deity was the only possible reason for suffering. When a poisonous snake bit the Apostle Paul, observers could only think of God's punishment. "And when the natives saw the creature hanging from his hand, they began saying to one another, 'Undoubtedly this man is a murderer...justice has not allowed him to live'" (Acts 28:4). The typical Jewish perspective on suffering was the same as that of the pagan. When Christ's disciples saw a blind man, they asked, "Rabbi, who sinned, this man or his parents, that he should be born blind?" (John 9:2). The Lord Jesus Christ responded from a completely different framework, giving a new concept of "no-fault" suffering. "Jesus answered, 'It was neither that this man sinned, nor his parents'" (John 9:3). In other words, the idea that suffering comes only from God's anger due to an individual's sin is far too narrow. While this can be the case, there also are many other causes and purposes for God allowing suffering. I would not presume to play the role of God the Holy Spirit and delineate to you God's purpose in your life, but you should consider all of the reasons the Bible gives for suffering. God wants us to confess our genuine sins, but there need not be a serious sin behind a particular hardship.

1. *Suffering destroys the illusion of self-sufficiency and drives us to dependence upon God.*

    • And He humbled you and let you be hungry, and fed you with manna which you did not know, nor did your fathers know, that He might make you understand that man does not live by bread alone, but man lives by everything that proceeds out of the mouth of the LORD (Deut. 8:3).

    • And because of the surpassing greatness of the revelations, for this reason, to keep me from exalt-ing myself, there was given me a thorn in the flesh, a messenger of Satan to buffet me - to keep me from exalting myself! .... And He has said to me, "My grace is sufficient for you, for power is per-fected in weakness," Most gladly, therefore, I will rather boast about my weaknesses, that the power of Christ may dwell in me (2 Cor. 12:7 and 9).

God allowed the Exodus generation to experience material deprivations so that they would learn the value of dependence upon God. God allowed the Apostle Paul to have some physical problem (a thorn in the flesh) to reduce pride and keep him in a state of dependence upon Himself. God used Paul greatly because Paul's weakness made him depend upon God.

Humans tend to forget about any need for God when life goes well. We live from paycheck to paycheck on a mundane level and act as if we do not need a spiritual dimension. Suffering changes that narrow vision. We realize our deep need. We can feel that we swim in the deep end of the lake with no hope of permanent human help. Often grief drives a person to faith in Christ for salvation. If it were not for suffering, the same person might never see the need for a Savior. Problems also drive those who are already Christians to a deeper level of dependence upon Christ. "When I am afraid, I will put my trust in Thee" (Psalm 56:3). Christian living, Christian growth, and Christian service begin when a believer realizes a deep dependence upon God for wisdom and strength.

Dependency upon God is one great blessing that arises from suffering. I hope your pain drives you to a sense of deep need for God. My family's experience with schizophrenia reminds me of Peter's question, "Lord, to whom shall we go? You have the words of eternal life" (John 6:68). When Peter learned that there was no other hope, answer, or alternative except dependence upon Christ, then God could use him greatly. This leads to a second purpose in suffering.

2. *Suffering makes us sympathetic and gives us credibility in ministry to others.*

> • Blessed be the God and Father of our Lord Jesus Christ, the Father of mercies and God of all comfort; who comforts us in all our affliction so that we may be able to comfort those who are in any affliction with the comfort with which we ourselves are comforted by God (2 Cor. 1:3-4).

I will never view those with a mental illness the way I did before my brother suffered from schizophrenia. Without suffering we might tend to be cold or dismiss the problems of the weak. The grief experience creates sensitivity and compassion. If you have a relative or friend with schizophrenia, you probably have a much greater love for all others with the disorder than would ever be possible without sharing in such grief.

Furthermore, suffering gives credibility in ministry to others. Often a pastor hears the quip, "You don't know what it is like." But pain gives a special preparation for ministry and insight about the needs of others. Sorrow serves as the engine of motivation. Grief gives unqualified credibility in ministry to others. **When we have suffered, we do know what it is like!**

Perhaps God has permitted your suffering to give you sympathy, motivation, and compassion for helping other families in their ordeals with mental illness. Go for it. Suffering is a terrible thing to waste.

3. *Suffering creates unity.*

I grew up in a wonderful church. Still, a church is not heaven. All churches have a share of petty jealousy, gossip, and bickering over trivialities. One icy February night, a carload of church members slipped across the median line and met a truck. A following carload of members stopped along the highway to help and never recognized the distorted bodies of their dear friends. We lost a youth group leader and his wife, our organist, a board member, and a Sunday school teacher. We gained instant church unity!

From the perspective of a tragedy, non-essential differences melt away. Most conflicts appear trivial. People usually rally around those most afflicted and pull together.

Ignorance and prejudice blunt this tendency to unite around the families of persons with mental illness. Never-theless, from God's perspective one of the purposes for allowing any tragedy is that it unites His children. Schizophrenia belongs in the tragic category no less than car accidents, miscarriages, other medical crises, fires, floods or tornadoes.

I hope your church will be knowledgeable enough and sensitive enough to "weep with those who weep" (Rom. 12:15) over schizophrenia. If not, take upon yourself the ministry of education. Learn about schizophrenia and share this information and experience with friends at church. With a better understanding you will find most of them will unite with you to give much needed compassion and support. At the very least, your suffering will cause a deep unity with other families facing the same heartbreak. God will use your grief to unite you with people you would have otherwise never met. He has worked this way in my life.

- ... that there should be no division in the body, but that the members should have the same care for one another. And if one member suffers, all the members suffer with it...(1 Cor. 12:25-26a).

4. *Suffering teaches us to pray.*

Every Christian would admit that a strong prayer life is desirable. Several Bible stories show us that we pray more when we face pressures. In Acts 12 wicked King Herod, the grandson of the Herod in the Christmas story, arrested the Apostle Peter with the intention of beheading him. How did the church respond to the pressure? "... prayer for him was being made fervently by the church to God" (Acts 12:5). Even the Lord Himself felt the stress of the impending cross and resorted to intense prayer.

And He went a little beyond them, and fell on His face and prayed, saying, "My Father, if it is possible, let this cup pass from Me; yet not as I will, but as Thou wilt" (Matt. 26:39).

Many believers, myself included, tend to be lazy in prayer when life is smooth. By contrast, we instinctively feel a need to pray when we face a crisis. The mental illness of a loved one may well result in a deeper prayer life.

5. *Suffering corrects priorities causing us to distinguish the eternal from the transitory, the important from the non-important.*

A TV commercial for athletic shoes blares, "Life is short. Play hard." A better Christian response would be, "Life is short. Live for Jesus now!" All serious diseases teach the fragility of physical life. Believers should praise God for their health (Ps. 103:1-3) and not take it for granted. The suffering of loved a loved one shows that there is no time to waste. We see that the time for action in service for the Lord Jesus Christ is now.

Many people live essentially selfish lives. Their goals lie in material acquisitions or only the pursuit of pleasure. Suffering gives us a more serious outlook on life. People are hurting, and soon this life will be past. Both truths are a basis for urgent work for Christ.

The Apostle Paul discovered that the trials of his life caused him to view life from an eternal perspective. Therefore, he valued work that had an eternal impact. Rather than live for material pursuits or selfish goals, he poured his life into service for God and ministry to spiritually needy people. Perhaps God has allowed your suffering to clarify your priorities. "Life is short. Live for Jesus now!"

- For momentary, light affliction is producing for us an eternal weight of glory far beyond all comparison, while we look not at the things which are seen, but at the things which are not seen; for the things which are seen are temporal, but the things which are not seen are eternal (2 Cor. 4:17-18).

- We must work the works of Him who sent Me, as long as it is day; night is coming, when no man can work (John 9:4).

6. *Suffering often leads to an increased witness.*

Our church received a letter from a Christian AIDS patient. She had innocently contracted AIDS from an unfaithful husband. She expected to die eventually, but in the meantime, she resolved that God had given her a platform to give the gospel. Many would listen to her story about Christ's grace and strength in facing death. Her sickness gave her opportunities to share the message of faith in Christ to people she would otherwise never influence. Jesus tells us Lazarus' suffering led to a greater glory for God. A later verse explains that Lazarus' painful experience caused many to believe in Christ.

> • But when Jesus heard it, He said, "This sickness is not unto death, but for the glory of God, that the Son of God may be glorified by it" (John 11:4). But the chief priests took counsel that they might put Lazarus to death also; because on account of him many of the Jews were going away, and were believing in Jesus (John 12:10-11).

A tragic illness for a family member or close friend can be a means for sharing the gospel with people who otherwise might never listen. A personal human-interest story that gives Christ credit for sustaining us during times of deep pain has a powerful impact upon others. There are few greater evidences of Christ's validity. We might think of the ministry of Joni Eareckson Tada, a Christian lady paralyzed from a sports accident. God has used her tragedy and disability to reach others with the gospel. Perhaps suffering in your family will put you in contact with those who need to trust in Christ as Savior. Maybe the plea to trust in Christ as Savior will sound credible coming from one who testifies that the Lord gives grace, courage, and strength in dealing with the pain of schizophrenia. Your grief qualifies you for a greater testimony, especially to the unsaved families of persons with mental illness. Some might otherwise never listen.

7. *Suffering teaches us the sanctity of life.*

In Matthew 25:40 the Lord refers to the "least of these my brethren." For our purposes it is not necessary to explain all the details of this phrase.[71] In reality Jesus does not view any as the "least". There used to be a societal agreement on the value of human life.

---

[71]In its context this phrase refers to the treatment of Jews during the future Tribulation period. Only genuine believers will protect the Jews from the end time tyrant, the Antichrist. Thus, Christ will see faith demonstrated by those who cared for His "brethren."

Unfortunately, America has divided over the sanctity of life. Some no longer value the unborn, the disabled, the elderly, the diseased. Yes, face the truth. Some place little value upon our family members who have schizophrenia. How else can we explain the lack of funding for research? What other opinion could explain cruel attitudes and practices toward the homeless with mental illness who lie in the streets?

A Christian who loves a relative or friend who has schizophrenia appreciates the value of all human life. Your suffering may motivate you to resist those who would destroy the sanctity of life ethic. Whether by public speaking, political activities, or ordinary conversation, your experiences with suffering will likely prompt you to be a voice for the innocent, a defense for the weak, and especially an advocate for consumer needs.

8.   *Suffering makes Christians more Christ-like.*

The Bible tells us that God the Father's will for God the Son involved **suffering, then glory.**[72]

- Was it not necessary for the Christ to suffer these things and to enter into His glory (Luke 24:26)?

- As to this salvation, the prophets who prophesied of the grace that would come to you made careful search and inquiry, seeking to know what person or time the Spirit of Christ within them was indicating as He predicted the sufferings of Christ and the glories to follow (1 Peter 1:10-11).

Your suffering over a loved one's schizophrenia can be used to increase Christ-likeness. Since God's plan is mysterious, I can only guess at the specifics. Perhaps you will have a deeper faith; more compassion; greater motivation for Christian service; a realization that heaven rather than earth is home; more credibility in witnessing; more

---

[72]Many Bible verses tell Christians to expect suffering. Some specifically give the pattern of suffering first and then glory (1 Peter 2:21, 5:1; Phil. 1:29; 1 Thess. 3:3; 2 Thess. 1:5). Although the Biblical author usually has persecution in mind, suffering from sickness could also produce the same spiritual effect in believers.

dependence upon God for courage, wisdom, and strength; a greater interest in the Scriptures; deeper prayer; more appreciation for the unity of Christian brothers; more holiness; or some other feature of Christ's rich character. You will have to ask God for the specific improvements He intends. Be confident that suffering, including grief over schizophrenia, is part of the process toward Christ-likeness and glory. If God's own Son did not escape hardship, we can hardly expect to escape. God's will for Jesus Christ was a mysterious process of suffering first and then glory.

Believers can expect the same pattern.

If you have never trusted in Christ, I guarantee that God allowed your suffering to awaken you to a need for the Savior. Jesus Christ, God the Son, paid for your sins on the cross and then defeated death by His resurrection. The Lord Jesus is trustworthy, ethical, and wise. He never told a lie, so it is reasonable to place faith in Him and His death on the cross. Salvation is not a matter of religious rituals or good deeds. A person becomes a Christian by faith in Christ.

- ...Believe in the Lord Jesus, and you shall be saved... (Acts 16:31).

The question "why" is a valid one. Those who value the Word of God have some clues as to why God allows suffering.

Suffering can produce limitations. Some with schizophrenia have reduced abilities to compete in a fast and demanding society. Yet, our society demands achievement. If we are really honest, most Americans base their whole self-esteem largely on their productivity or social standing. But do people not have value regardless of vocation, artistic or athletic talent? Do I have more value than my little pre-school daughter because I have academic degrees, but she has not yet been to kindergarten? Is my brother without worth because schizophrenia prohibits him from working? Although most Americans believe a sense of self-worth is essential, we can uncritically assume its primary source is achievement. This false assumption hurts all people and no group more than our relatives and friends with schizophrenia. Chapter Five will explain a better foundation for human value.

Questions and Thoughts to
Consider from Chapter Four

1. Have church members or ministers led you to believe that sin is the only basis for suffering?

2. Have you received any special comfort and support from church members or a minister?

3. Has your pain increased your sympathy for all others with struggles?

4. Has your suffering brought you together with new friends that you might not otherwise know or be able to help?

5. If 25-40% of all long-term hospital stays are for schizophrenia, why doesn't the public know more about the disorder and respond with greater efforts?

Chapter Five

The Source of Human Value

The Bible teaches that man has a dark side (Rom. 3:10,23). Read any metropolitan newspaper for confirmation. Nevertheless, the Biblical view of man also leads Christians to assert the immense value of every person. Christians through the centuries have made personal sacrifices to address spiritual, emotional, and physical needs because they believe in the dignity and worth of every person. This value exists prior to and independent of an individual's abilities.

Let us begin with the strong assertion that our relatives with schizophrenia possess infinite value. Yes, they have skills and achievements. We are grateful for the abilities they possess. It is wise to praise them and to draw attention to their abilities. This gives a secondary support for their sense of worth[73]. Nevertheless, they (like all humans) have inherent worth regardless of how they perform. Human value derives from what we are rather than from what we can do. Humans have worth because of how God views us and what He has done for us.

By God's evaluation, a homeless wanderer, or a mental hospital patient, or a prison inmate possesses the same value as the President, a physician, or a minister of a huge church. Several Biblical truths express the measureless worth of all people including non-Christians. Additional Biblical truths reinforce the worth of those who have trusted in Christ as Savior. Those who profess to be Christians should view people as Christ does. He extends grace, mercy, compassion, and unconditional love.

---

[73]Christ taught "without me you can do nothing" (John 15:5). However, a Christian may rejoice in what God has accomplished through him. "I can do all things through Christ who strengthens me" (Phil. 4:13). Sinful vanity arises if we boast of what we alone can do, but the Bible gives examples of Christians feeling satisfaction in what God has done through them. "I have fought the good fight..." (2 Tim. 4:7).

Value in All People

Almost everyone knows the Bible forbids cursing. This prohibition may seem quaint and old-fashioned in our generation, but consider the underlying reason.

> • With it [the tongue] we bless our Lord and Father; and with it we curse men, *who have been made in the likeness of God*; from the same mouth come both blessing and cursing. My brethren, these things ought not to be this way (James 3:9-10).

God prohibits cursing another human because it insults the value of that person. Every human possesses an image of God in the sense that he or she is an eternal being. God exists in eternity future. So will you and I. So will every person with schizophrenia. Christians, beginning with relatives, should view those with schizophrenia as valuable by virtue of possessing the image of God and being eternal souls. A second Bible teaching that proves the value of all people comes from the Old Testament. God has a personal concern for each individual.

> • Before I formed you in the womb I knew you... (Jer. 1:5)

All people have value because God was interested in us even before we were born. To God no person is just a faceless statistic. No human is just a case study for a research project or dissertation. To God people are not throw away circuit boards who get tossed out when they cannot keep up with the workload. He has a personal concern for everyone beginning before birth and extending throughout life. Those who have schizophrenia also have God's per-sonal attention. To Him they are not impersonal objects or curious freaks.

Finally, the unconditional love of Christ who paid for the sins of the entire world shows how much God values people. We have worth because the Lord Jesus Christ loved us enough to die for us on the cross.

> • For God so loved the world, that He gave His only begotten Son, that whoever believes in Him should not perish, but have eternal life (John 3:16).

- Greater love has no one than this, that one lay down his life for his friend (John.15:13).

Christ gave Himself in our place to pay for our sins so that those who believe in Him might be forgiven. Of course, not everyone appreciates what Christ has done or accepts Him as Savior. But the fact remains that every person has so much worth to God that he or she was worth the death of His beloved Son. Even though it must remain a mystery, God valued the human race enough to exchange His Son's life to rescue us. This proves our tremendous worth to God and ought to establish the conviction that Christians must value all people. Christ died for those with a mental illness, which proves that they are worth much to God. Therefore, we should also consider them to be precious. If Christian views of those with schizophrenia reflect God's views, then we will regard these people as eternal souls in the image of God, the recipients of God's personal concern, and the object of God's deepest and unconditional love. This holds true for all, even those who do not profess to be Christians.

Theological Truths Demonstrating the Value of Christians

My brother has trusted in Christ as His Savior. So have many other people with a schizophrenic disorder[74]. Those who doubt this are invited to speak with participants of the chapel services formerly conducted by the Panhandle Alliance for the Mentally Ill. These believers share equally with all other Christians in the blessings of faith. Several benefits to Christians reinforce their value before God. People like Mark should understand that despite having an infirmity that increases their spiritual struggles, God has credited them with Christ's righteousness, welcomed them as His children into His family, and gifted them for service. Christians should take all of these truths into account as we view other believers with schizophrenia. Blessings

---

[74]Dr. Robert Lightner's work *Heaven for Those Who Can't Believe* dis-cusses the doctrine of salvation relative to infants and those mentally unable to understand faith. Robert P. Lightner. *Heaven for Those Who Can't Believe.* Schaumburg, IL: Regular Baptist Press, 1977. Welch gives hope by relating a story of a woman with Alzheimer's who trusted in Christ during a lucid period before relapsing. Edward T. Welch, *Counselor's Guide to the Brain and Its Disorders*, 115.

arising from Christ's work on the cross provide a great foundation to teach mentally ill believers their self-worth.

One aspect of the cross involves Christ's taking our sins in the sense that He legally paid for them and satisfied God's justice. The corresponding truth is that those who believe are credited with Christ's perfect and eternal righteousness. This also satisfies God's justice. Christ took our sins. He gives His righteousness to those who trust Him as Savior. Relative to God's role as judge, a believer legally stands before God as blameless and uncondemned. Christ's righteousness is *our* righteousness.

> He made Him who knew no sin to be sin on *our* behalf, that *we* might become the righteousness of God in Him (2 Cor. 5:21). Theology affects life. If anything ought to make a person feel worth, it would be the idea that he stands before God, the Judge, with all the perfection of Jesus Christ. My brother, like all Christians, has been clothed in Christ's righteousness.[75] Relative to God's justice, Mark stands uncondemned, acquitted, and vindicated. If the truth of justification by faith does not prove human worth, then nothing else can.[76] Mark might not understand the theology, but he can understand that God as a judge holds no anger toward him and that he need not fear any condemnation (see John 5:24; Rom. 8:1).

A second truth would be more easily understood. All believers are the children of God. All will share in Christ's glory in an eternal heaven.

> • But as many as received Him, to them He gave the right to become children of God, even to those who believe in His name (John 1:12).

---

[75]See Isaiah 61:10.

[76]The doctrine of justification by faith was a major point in the Protestant Reformation. All Protestant denominations originally believed this doctrine. The evangelical wing of all denominations still does.

- The Spirit Himself bears witness with our spirit that we are children of God, and if children, heirs also, heirs of God and fellow heirs with Christ, if indeed we suffer with Him in order that we may also be glorified with Him (Rom. 8:16-17).

It is impossible to put a price on my children's value to me. God feels the same way about those who trust Christ. That includes the ones with schizophrenia. They share in that lofty status of being part of God's family. That is how other Christians should view them. With careful teaching they can share in the sense of value that comes from knowing one is a child of God.[77]

Finally, believers should possess a sense of worth arising from God's desire for them to serve others. The Bible teaches that every believer has a contribution to make to God's work in this world. Every believer is a minister in a generic sense. The Scripture does not exclude those with schizophrenia from having spiritual gifts that equip them for Christian ministry.

- As each one has received a special gift, employ it in serving one another, as good stewards of the manifold grace of God (1 Peter 4:10).

Let no one think that people with a mental illness are incapable of ministry. I have seen consumers lead singing, read the Bible, pray, and recite poems they have written, as well as, perform skits and plays. They ministered by sharing themselves in ways that often excel the typical church member. Being accustomed to group meetings, they often reveal themselves with a transparency and honesty usually not found in an average church congregation. They can offer touching prayer requests that show sincerity. After a sermon, one consumer suggested that we should pray that "we will do what we have heard". I wish all Christians felt that way. I think I have ministered to their

---

[77]To say a believer is a child or son of God does not mean we are sons of God in the same sense that Jesus Christ is the "Son of God." The Apostle John distinguishes Christ's Sonship from a believer's sonship with the assertion that Christ is "the only begotten Son". His Sonship is unique. Paul's way of making the same distinction is to compare Christians to adopted sons and Christ to a natural Son. Christ's Sonship involves being God the Son, co-equal with the Father (Rom. 8:14-16).

needs, but I know they have ministered to me by making me more tender and compassionate. The special battles these fellow Christians have (see Chapter Two pp.39-40) can teach lessons to other Christians about our own moral struggles. I honestly believe there are some spiritual lessons that only those with schizophrenia can teach the Church in general. Also, their hardship gives them special credibility in ministry to unbelievers with schizophrenia. God wants those with schizophrenia to serve Him. The rest of us should rejoice in the sense of worth consumers can share by being a part of His work.

The same truths that establish the worth of all people confirm the worth of people with schizophrenia. They possess God's image with eternal souls. God has a personal interest in them, and Christ regarded them as precious enough to die for them.

The same truths that establish the worth of Christians confirm the worth of believers who have schizophrenia. Having been justified by faith, they have a perfect legal standing before God as judge. Christ took their sins and credits them with His righteousness. They are children of God who will share in heaven. They have spiritual gifts that enable them to make contributions to God's work. In some ways these are contributions only they can make.

Human value comes less from what we do than how God views us and what He has done for us. Regardless of any limitations, those with schizophrenia have worth to God. They have value to their families. The Church as a whole should minister to and embrace them and their families since they are just as important as any other subculture.

Our next and final chapter should help toward this goal of increasing ministry to families and consumers by clearing up confusion on the differences between demon influence and schizophrenia. Confusion over this issue can needlessly hinder efforts to embrace both people with schizophrenia and their relatives.

Questions and Thoughts to Consider from Chapter Five

1. Do you agree or disagree that the primary basis for human value does not lie in performance?

2. Can you see dangers (or benefits) in teaching children to rest their self-esteem on achievement?

3. Explain the differences between "without Me you can do nothing" and "I can do all things through Christ who strengthens me".

4. How does the theology of "justification by faith" change the way we view self, other Christians, and believers with schizophrenia?

5. Can the idea of being a "child of God be taught to Christians with schizophrenia without bringing confusion? Would this help them feel worth?

Chapter Six

Differentiation of Schizophrenia
From Demon Influence

Every Christian who researches schizophrenia wonders about the demonic. The New Testament mentions demons over 100 times. All New Testament authors, except the writer of Hebrews, teach about demons. Jesus Christ gives the most credible evidence for the existence and power of demons. He conversed with them (Matt. 8:29). He gave His disciples power over them (Matt. 10:1ff.). He called the devil "the ruler of this world" (John 16:11). Adherents to Christ's authority will believe in the existence of demons.

American society has transformed its views on the supernatural in the last generation. More and more people are open to the supernatural. While many still reject the reality of demons, good empirical evidence exists to con-firm the supernatural. It is a mistake to dismiss either Biblical authority or valid observations about occultic activity.

David W. Van Gelder, Ph.D., tells of an account of demon possession in South Carolina. The group of people witnessing the seizure included two medical doctors, one psychologist, one professor of pastoral counseling, one minister, and three seminary students. Van Gelder writes of a young man on "all fours snarling like an animal".[78] A crucifix fell to the floor, and nails in the wall melted. The boy cursed in another voice which spoke through him. His writhing on the floor stopped only when he prayed to trust in Christ. Although these witnesses were not inclined to accept an occultic explanation for the phenomena, the terrible ordeal forced them to this conclusion. Dr. Van Gelder analyzed his experience in a 1987 article in *The Journal of Pastoral Care.*

The second possibility [that it was only a psychotic or epileptic experience] assumes ignorance on the part of the

---

[78]David W. Van Gelder, "A Case of Demon Possession," *Journal of Pastoral Care*, 41(2) (1987):151.

participants. It is an option that has been pressed on me several times since that evening. But I have seen rolandic, petit mal and grand mal seizures. I have seen various psychoses, psychotic breaks and a variety of organic syndromes. I have worked in a maximum-security unit for the criminally insane. Even if I do not know what I saw, I know what I did not see. It was none of the above. Besides that, other professional counselors were there as well. We are not speaking of isolated observations and analysis... The time has come, however, when we can no longer relegate these experiences simply to the field of psychology. Psychologists themselves are beginning to question the phenomena and are looking for new frames of reference. We need to supplement the ancient conceptions of demonic activity in the personal spiritual world with modern understandings of personality theory and its appropriate techniques for healing.[79]

T. Craig Isaacs did some fascinating research on demon possession for his doctoral dissertation at the California School of Professional Psychology in Berkeley. His research question was, "Is possession a phenomena independent of the current commonly accepted psychodiagnostic categories?"[80] Isaacs submitted to five experienced psychodiagnosticians 14 cases of those certified by the Episcopal Church as demon possessed. They examined the people to "assess the applicability of the diagnostic categories of the current *Diagnostic and Statistical Manual III* to each of the cases...."[81] The study concludes that possession is unlike any of the other established categories of mental illness. Isaacs writes:

Is possession a phenomenon independent of the current commonly accepted psychodiagnostic categories? The answer from all three areas indicates that it is.... Therefore, certain psychological researchers began to turn their attention to possession as a distinct phenomenon. Pattison felt that rather than

---

[79]Ibid., 158-159.

[80]Craig T. Isaacs, "The Possessive States Disorder: The Diagnosis of Demonic Possession," *Pastoral Psychology*, 35(4) (1987): 264.

[81]Ibid.

approaching possession with the disease-oriented models of medicine, research should turn to a culturally-minded model, thus leaning back on the data being gathered by the anthropologists. Henderson began to warn researchers of attempting to merely fit possession into one of the current diagnostic categories. He states that "a well known pitfall of scholarly endeavor is our propensity to dogmatize those theoretical postulates which are currently in vogue. It is accordingly fashionable at least in professional circles to dismiss the notions of possession and exorcism as outmoded medieval superstitions of, at best, historical interest. Such a dismissal would be decidedly premature." Recently another psychiatrist, Scott Peck, has broken on the scene with the assertion that demonic possession should be accepted on its own merits, and that psychiatry and psychology must begin to take seriously the active presence of evil in the lives of patients.[82]

Humanists/atheists who deny the supernatural do so against valid Biblical and experiential evidence to the contrary. However, even those who choose to remain skeptical still must relate to Christians who believe very much in the supernatural.[83] Many Christians who endure a family member's battle with schizophrenia will have questions about

---

[82]Ibid., 264-266.

[83]I appreciate the comments of Dr. LeRoy Spaniol on the value of religion in helping families in distress. Therapists may not share Christian faith, but they should respect a Christian family's beliefs as helpful to that family. Just as I appealed in Lesson Two for ministers to see limited value in the psychiatric profession even when they cannot agree with everything, I would hope non-Christian psychiatrists and psychologists could see some value in pastoral care. When families have theological concerns, what is wrong with referrals to clergy? "Family members who are religious also take care of themselves through prayer, Bible reading, and fellowship with other believers. Religious beliefs and activities can sustain family members in their caring. Acceptance is often fostered by deep religious beliefs.... Religious beliefs imply that there is more to life than what we ordinarily see, and that there is a power and a force that supports us if we are open to acknowledging it and calling upon it. Family members report strong religious beliefs and regularly acknowledge that these beliefs sustain them in their daily lives." LeRoy Spaniol, "Coping Strategies of Family Caregivers" in *Families of the Mentally Ill: Coping and Adaptation,* edited by Agnes B. Hatfield and Harriet Lefley (New York: The Guilford Press, 1987), 214.

demon involvement. I did, especially when I saw my brother ripping up a Bible and smashing Christian wall decorations. Those who worry about demonic involvement with a loved one deserve real answers instead of a condescending response that dismisses such concern as nonsense on the part of ignorant people. The complete topic of pastoral care for the demon-possessed is not germane to this study, but readers may find reassurance by an explanation of differences between schizophrenia and demon possession.[84]

The Bible itself makes a distinction between disease and possession (see Mark 6:13). Thus, Christian theology should recognize the difference between organic brain disorder and demonic control. At least six factors differentiate schizophrenia from demon possession as described in the Bible. These have helped me better understand by brother's illness.

1. *Attraction to vs. Aversion to Religion*

Mallard Sall, a psychiatrist from Anaheim, California, makes this observation.

> Demons want nothing to do with Christ. Conversely, people who are deeply mentally disturbed are often devoutly religious. Unlike demons, they want to be close to Jesus or have some kind of deep religious experience.[85]

Alfred Lechler, a German psychiatrist, reaches the same conclusion.

> Furthermore, if he displays no signs of opposition to any form of Christian counseling, or just listens indifferently and remains unmoved when people attempt to exorcise demons, or

---

[84]For a more complete study I have written a paper called, "Demons and Pastoral Care" presented in doctoral work at Dallas Theological Seminary. A minister should never diagnose the presence of the demonic unless the overt characteristics in the New Testament are present.

[85]Mallard J. Sall, "Demon Possession or Psychology? A Critical Differentiation," *Journal of Psychology and Theology*, 4(4) (1976): 288.

if he finds no difficulty in pronouncing the name of Jesus, all this is indicative of mental illness rather than the demonic.[86]

Ronald Koteskey, a psychology professor at Asbury College, agrees with their conclusions.[87]

I have visited in mental hospitals enough to know that many patients desire religious instruction. The Texas Panhandle Alliance for the Mentally Ill initiated the idea of chapel services for our group. Many consumers show interest in Jesus Christ. By contrast we know from the New Testament that demons hate any involvement with the things of Christ.

2. *Irrational Speech vs. Rational Speech*

In New Testament accounts involving demons, the demons spoke in a rational manner. *Untreated* people with schizophrenia will often speak in nonsense and jump rapidly between unrelated topics. My brother does this.

The fact that the demons spoke in a rational manner is a third distinction... They communicated in a rational manner. They... spoke clearly with purpose and meaning, possessing the ability to carry on a real dialogue. The speech and logical process of the schizophrenic are often incoherent. They produce "word salads" and irrationalities that do not make sense, in contrast to the speech behavior of demons.[88]

A possessed person is in fact mentally healthy in spite of the fact that at intervals he may exhibit certain symptoms of

---

[86]Kurt Koch and Alfred Lechler, *Occult Bondage and Deliverance* (Grand Rapids: Kregal Publications, 1970), 162.

[87]Ronald C. Koteskey, "Toward the Development of a Christian Psychology: Adjustment and Maladjustment," *Journal of Psychology and Theology*, 7 (3) (Fall 1979): 182.

[88]Sall, "Demon Possesion or Psychopathology?", 288.

mental abnormalities .... Moreover the words the mentally ill person hears are often completely nonsensical.[89]

In such cases where the voices make sense (not nonsense as in the case of schizophrenia, a condition of chemical imbalance in the brain)... We should strongly suspect demonic forces...[90]

3. *Ordinary Learning vs. Supernatural Knowledge*

Demons in the New Testament would speak through people to convey knowledge that otherwise could not have been known to the possessed individuals. Those with a mental illness have no such ability to know facts that they have not acquired by normal means of learning. Koch states,

For example, clairvoyance itself is never a sign of mental illness, and a mental patient will never be able to speak in a voice or a language he has previously not learned.[91]

4. *Normal vs. Occultic Phenomena*

There is an aspect to demon activity that is just plain spooky. If there are occurrences of poltergeists, levitations, trances, telepathy (and these cannot be ruled out as being optical illusions or fraudulent displays), then one is not dealing with "ordinary" schizophrenia.[92] These "most dramatic aspects," that were "frequently encountered" helped stump Isaac's panel of psychodiagnosticians at Berkeley.[93] He lists the following as indications of possession as opposed to mental illness:

---

[89]Koch and Lechler, *Occult Bondage and Deliverance*, 162-163.

[90]C. Fred Dickason, Demon *Possession and the Christian* (Westchester, IL: Crossway Books, 1987) 228.

[91]Koch and Lechler, *Occult Bondage and Deliverance*, 58.

[92]Henry and Mary Virkler, "Demonic Involvement in Human Life and Illness," *Journal of Psychology and Theology*, 5(2) (1977): 100.

[93]Isaacs, *The Possessive States Disorder*, 269.

.... some form of paranormal phenomena, such as poltergeist-type phenomena, telepathy, levitation or strength out of proportion to age. There is an impact on others: paranormal phenomena, stench, coldness or the feeling of an alien presence or that the patient has lost a human quality, is experienced by someone other than the patient.[94]

5. *The Claim to be Possessed*

Authors who have clinical experience both with demon possession and mental illness believe those who claim to be possessed are very likely **not possessed**. Demons wish to be secretive and do not voluntarily claim to be present. Lechler writes:

While the mental patient will speak in extravagant tones of the demons he alleges to be living within, the possessed person avoids all mention of demons as long as no one approaches him on a spiritual level.[95]

6. *The Effects of Therapy*

If prayer solves the problem, then it was probably not schizophrenia. If medicine helps alleviate the problem, it was not demon possession. Demons cannot be exorcised by phenothiazine, antidepressant drugs, or E.C.T.[96]

Hallucinations are cured by psychological treatment, while demon possession can be cured only by prayer and fasting as Christ indicated.[97]

---

[94]Ibid., 272.

[95]Koch and Lechler, *Occult Bondage and Deliverance*, 162.

[96]Walter Johnson, "Demon Possession and Mental Illness," *Journal of the American Scientific Affiliation*, 34(3) (1982): 151.

[97]Sall, *Demon Possession or Psychopathology?*, 289.

I discovered that all of the "demons" I was seeing were allergic to Thorazine and that, in nearly every case, a week or two on Thorazine made the "demons" go away...[98]

Christian families of those with carefully diagnosed schizophrenia need not worry about demon involvement. Furthermore, they need not feel the pressure of well- meaning relatives or friends who suggest demons as the primary explanation for the strange behavior that accompanies schizophrenia. The Bible never presents a case of demon possession where anyone had the slightest trouble recognizing the presence of demons. It was such a strange, terrifying and overtly supernatural experience that everyone involved knew demons were present: Christ, the Apostles, Jewish religious leaders and common people. No other conclusion was possible. Unless a case closely parallels the New Testament description of demon possession, the church and the family should regard it as they would a chronic, severe and baffling sickness. Ministers need a deeper knowledge about schizophrenia, but many skills in ministry relative to diseases in general also apply to families of the mentally ill (and often to consumers after they have had medical treatment).

Conclusion

Families of those with schizophrenia face many problems that are not within the domain of spiritual care. They want to know about medicine, housing, social security, estate planning, and the practical knowledge needed to communicate and live with a mentally ill person. Professionals in secular disciplines can give them advice in these areas. However, Christians have an important contribution to make in ministry to these hurting families in areas beyond secular psychiatry and social work. Once the true nature of schizophrenia is understood (Chapter Two), Christians can give much guidance to families and consumers. The Bible gives help for all of the painful emotional responses of the families of the mentally ill (Chapter Three). The Bible gives a theology of suffering whereas psychology alone has no explanation (Chapter Four). The Word of God insists on the value of every human even when there are limitations in performance (Chapter

---

[98]Danny Korem and Paul Meier, *The Fakers* (Grand Rapids: Baker Book House, 1980), 160.

Five). Furthermore, educated ministers should be able to answer questions relative to schizophrenia and demons (Chapter Six).

Secular books on mental illness often recommend that a family turn to a minister or church family for support. The value of that advice depends upon the knowledge and character of a particular minister or church. Whatever flaws exist in the church's response to schizophrenia they do not arise from deficiencies in God or the Scriptures. The Bible has truths that minister to the needs of families of people who have the schizophrenia disorder.

Hopefully, the future will see greater sensitivity to these hurting people, and evangelicals will learn how to better serve them. I pray that these studies have helped you and will lead to improvement in ministry within that great family composed of everyone who has faith in Jesus Christ as Savior.

Questions and Thoughts to Consider From Chapter Six

1. Has anyone actually told you that demons caused your family member's mental illness?

2. Does your family member express interest in spiritual concerns? Does the state hospital have a chaplain? Could your local Alliance for the Mentally Ill find a Bible-believing minister who is interested in helping?

Mental Health Organizations

Alzheimer's Association – www.alz.org
225 N. Michigan Avenue, Floor 17
Chicago, Illinois 60601
(800) 272-3900

NAMI (National Alliance for the Mentally Ill) www.nami.org
2107 Wilson Blvd Suite 300
Arlington, VA 22201
(703) 524-7600

Texas Alliance for the Mentally Ill – www.namitexas.org
Affiliate of National Alliance for the Mentally Ill
Fountain Park Plaza III, 2800 South IH35, Suite 140
Austin, TX 78704
(512) 693-2000 / (800) 633-3760

National Depressive and Manic Depressive Association www.ndma.org
730 N. Franklin St. Suite 501
Chicago, IL 60610
(312) 642-7243 / (800) 826-3632

Christian Clinics/Hospitals

Rapha - Hospital Treatment Centers - www.rapha.info
3021 Gateway Drive Suite 290
Irving, TX 75063
1-800-383-HOPE

Minirth-Meier Clinic
1200 E. Collins Blvd., Suite 300
Richardson, TX 75081
1-972 669-1733 / 1-800 646-4784

BIBLIOGRAPHY

A. Books

Abramson, Nancy S., Jean K. Quam, and Mona Wasow, editors. *The Elderly and Chronic Mental Illness*. New Directions for Mental Health Services. ed. H.Richard Lamb. San Francisco: Jossey-Bass, Inc., Publishers, 1986.

A *Family Affair: Helping Families Cope With Mental Illness*. New York: Brunner/Mazel Publishers, 1986.

Andreasen, Nancy. *The Broken Brain: The Biological Revolution in Psychiatry*. New York: Harper and Row, 1984.

Bennett, George. *When the Mental Patient Comes Home*. Wayne Oates, ed. Philadelphia: Westminster Press, 1980.

Bernheim, Kayla F. and Anthony F. Lehman. *Working with Families of the Mentally Ill*. New York: W.W. Norton and Company, 1985.

Bernheim, K.F., Richard R. Lewine, and Caroline T. Beale. *The Caring Family Living with Chronic Mental Illness*. New York: Random House, Publishers, 1982.

Bobgan, Martin and Deidre Bobgan. *Psychoheresy*. Santa Barbara, CA: East Gate Publishers, 1987.

Boisen, Anton T. *Out of the Depths: An Autobiographical Study of Mental Disorder and Religious Experience*. New York: Harper and Row, 1960.

Bruden, Ernest E. *Ministering to Deeply Troubled People*. EngleWood Cliffs, N.J.: Prentice Hall, 1963.

Burch, Claire, *Stranger in the Family: A Guide to Living with the Emotionally Disturbed*. Indianapolis and New York: the Bobbs Merrill Company, Inc., 1972.

Clinebell, Howard. *Basic Types of Pastoral Care and Counseling.* Rev. ed. Nashville: Abingdon Press, 1984.

Clinebell, Howard J., ed. *Community Mental Health: The Role of Church and Temple.* Nashville: Abingdon Press, 1970.

Clinebell, Howard John. *The Mental Health Ministry of the Local Church.* reprinted. Nashville: Abingdon Press, 1975.

Collins, Gary. *Can You Trust Psychology?* Downers Grove, IL: Inter Varsity Press, 1988.

Collins, Gary. *Christian Counseling: A Comprehensive Guide.* Rev. ed. Dallas: Word Publishers, 1988.

Collins, Gary. *Fractured Personalities: The Psychology of Mental Illness.* Carol Stream, IL: Creation House, 1972.

Cosgrove, Mark P. *The Essence of Human Nature.* Grand Rapids: Zondervan and Probe, 1977.

Cosgrove, Mark P. and James D. Mallory with a response by O. Quentin Hyder. *Mental Health: A Christian Approach.* Grand Rapids: Zondervan Publishing House, 1977.

Davis, Robert. *My Journey into Alzheimer's Disease: Helpful Insights for Family and Friends.* Wheaton, IL: Tyndale House Publishers, Inc., 1989.

Deutsch, Albert. *The Mentally Ill in America.* Rev. ed. New York: Columbia University Press, 1947.

Dickason, Fred C. *Demon Possession and the Christian.* Westchester, IL: Crossway Books, 1987.

Edwards, Henry. *What Happened To My Mother (Not To Mention the Rest of Us)?* New York: Harper & Row, 1981.

Fish, Sharon. *Alzheimer's Caring For Your Loved One, Caring For Yourself.* Batavia, IL: Lion Publishing Corporation, 1990.

Garcia, Juan. *Learning More About Attention Deficit Disorders.* Dallas: Rapha Publishing, 1991.

Gottesman, Irving I. *Schizophrenia Genesis: The Origins of Madness.* New York: W.H. Freeman and Company, 1991.

Hart, Arcibald D., Gary L. Gulbranson, and Jim Smith, *Mastering Pastoral Counseling.* Portland, Oregon: Multnomah Press and Christianity Today Inc., 1992.

Hatfield, Agnes B. *Family Education in Mental Illness.* New York: The Guilford Press, 1990.

Hatfield, Agnes B. and Harriet P. Lefley, eds. *Families of the Mentally Ill: Coping and Adaptation.* New York: The Guilford Press, 1987.

Hatfield, Agnes B. editor. *Families of the Mentally Ill: Meeting the Challenges.* New Directions for Mental Health Services, ed. H. Richard Lamb. San Francisco: Josey-Bass Publishers, 1986.

Jeffries, J.J. et al. *Living and Working with Schizophrenia.* Second ed. Toronto: University of Toronto Press, 1990.

Johnson, Julie Tallard. *Hidden Victims: An Eight-Stage Healing Process For Families and Friends of the Mentally Ill.* New York: Doubleday, 1988.

Jones, Stanton L. and Richard E. Butman. *Modern Psychotherapies.* Downers Grove, IL: InterVarsity Press, 1991.

Kelsey, Morton T. *Psychology, Medicine, and Christian Healing.* Rev. ed. San Francisco: Harper and Row Publications, 1988.

Kilpatrick, William Kirk. *Psychological Seduction: The Failure of Modern Psychology.* Nashville: Thomas Nelson Publishers, 1983.

Knight, Ward A. *My Church was a Mental Hospital*. Philadelphia: United Church Press, 1974.

Koch, Kurt E. and Alfred Lechler. *Occult Bondage and Deliverance*. Reprint edition. Grand Rapids: Kregel Publications, 1970.

Korem, Danny,and Paul Meier. *The Fakers*. Grand Rapids: Baker Book House, 1980.

Korpell, Herbert S. *How You Can Help: A Guide For Families of Psychiatric Hospital Patients*. American Psychiatric Press, 1984.

Lefley, Harriet P., and Dale L. Johnson. *Families as Allies in the Treatment of the Mentally Ill*. Washington, D.C.: American Psychiatric Press, 1990.

Lightner, Robert. *Heaven For Those Who Cannot Believe*. Schaumberg, IL: Regular Baptist Press, 1977.

Little, Gilbert L. and Theodore H. Epp. *The Christian and Emotional Problems*. Lincoln, NE: Back to the Bible Broadcasting, 1970.

Lutzer, Erwin. *Managing Your Emotions*. Wheaton, IL: Victor Books, 1983.

Mace, Nancy L., and Peter V. Rabins. *The 36 Hour Day: A Family Guide to Caring for Persons with Alzheimer's Disease*. New York: Warner Books, 1981.

Martindale, Don and Edith Martindale. *Mental Disability in America Since World War II*. New York: Philosophical Library, 1985.

Meier, Paul D., Frank B. Minrith, Frank B. Wichern, and Donald E. Ratcliff. *Introduction to Psychology and Counseling: Christian Perspectives and Applications*. Reprinted. Grand Rapids: Baker Book House, 1991.

Mendel, Werner. *Treating Schizophrenia.* San Francisco: Josey-Bass Publishers, 1989.

Menninger, Karl. *Whatever Became of Sin?* reprint edition. New York: Bantam Books, 1978.

Miller, William R. and Kathleen A. Jackson. *Practical Psychology for Pastors.* Englewood Cliffs, NJ: Prentice-Hall, Inc., 1985.

Minirth, Frank. *Christian Psychiatry.* Old Tappan, NJ: Fleming H. Revel Co., 1977.

Minirth, Frank B., and Paul D. Meier. *Happiness Is A Choice.* Grand Rapids: Baker Book House, 1978.

Minirth, Frank B., Paul D. Meier and Kevin Kinback. *Ask the Doctors: Questions and Answers from "The Minrith-Meier Clinic" Broadcast.* Grand Rapids: Baker Book House, 1991.

Narramore, Clyde M. *The Psychology of Counseling.* Grand Rapids: Zondervan Publishing House, 1961.

Oates, Wayne E. *Pastoral Counseling.* Philadelphia: The Westminster Press, 1974.

Oates, Wayne. *The Religious Care of the Psychiatric Patient.* Philadelphia: Westminster Press, 1978.

Papolos, Demitri and Janice Papolos. *Overcoming Depression.* New York: Harper Perennial, 1988.

Park, Clara Clairborne with Leon N. Shapiro. *You Are Not Alone: Understanding and Dealing with Mental Illness - A Guide for Patients, Families, Doctors, and Other Professionals.* Boston: Little, Brown, and Company, 1976.

Powell, Lenore S., and Katie Courtice. *Alzheimer's Disease: A Guide for Families.* Reading, MD: Addison-Wesley Publishing, 1983.

Rushford, Patricia. *The Help,Hope and Cope Book for People with Aging Parents*. Old Tappan, NJ: Fleming H. Revell Co., 1985.

Safford, Florence. *Caring For the Mentally Impaired Elderly: A Family Guide*. New York: Henry Holt and Company, 1986.

Sheehan, Susan. *Is There No Place on Earth For Me?* Boston:Houghton Mifflin Co., 1982.

Shelly, Judith Allen, Sandra D. John and Others. *Spiritual Dimensions of Mental Health*. Downers Grove, IL: Inter-Varsity Press, 1983.

Sheridan, Carmel. *Failure Free Activities For the Alzheimer's Patient: A Guidebook for Caregivers*. Oakland, CA: Cottage Books, 1987.

Smith, Nancy Covert. *Of Pebbles and Pearls*. Waco,TX: Word Books, 1974.

Southard, Samuel. *The Family and Mental Illness*. Philadelphia: Westminster Press, 1957.

Spotts, Steven W. *Learning More About Depression*. Dallas: Rapha Publishing, 1991.

Torrey E. Fuller. *Freudian Fraud: The Malignant Effect of Freud's Theory on American Thought and Culture*. New York: Harper-Collins, 1992.

Torrey, E. Fuller. *Nowhere to Go: The Tragic Odyssey of the Homeless Mentally Ill*. New York: Harper and Row, 1989.

Torrey, E. Fuller. *Surviving Schizophrenia: A Family Manual*. Rev. ed. New York: Harper and Row, 1988.

Treffert, Donald A. *Extraordinary People: Understanding Idiot Savants*. New York: Harper and Row, 1989.

Walsh, Maryellen. *Schizophrenia: Straight Talk for Families and Friends*. Reprint ed. New York: Warner Books, 1985.

Watson, Tom Jr., and Stan Schmidt. *Holding God Hostage.* Brentwood, TN: Woldemuth and Hyatt Publishers, 1991.

Welch, Edward T. *Counselors Guide to the Brain and Its Disorders.* Grand Rapids: Zondervan Publishing Co., 1991.

White, John. *Putting the Soul Back in Psychology: When Secular Values Ignore Spiritual Realities.* Downers Grove, IL: Inter-Varsity Press, 1987.

White, Robin. *The Special Child: A Parent's Guide to Mental Disabilities.* Boston: Little, Brown, and Co., 1978.

Wilson, Louise. *This Stranger, My Son.* New York: G.P. Putman's Sons, 1968.

Wise, Carroll A. *Psychiatry and the Bible.* New York: Harper and Row, 1956.

Wood, Garth. *The Myth of Neurosis.* New York: Harper and Row Publishers, 1986.

Yancy, Philip. *Where Is God When It Hurts?* Grand Rapids: Zondervan Publishing House, 1977.

B. Periodicals, Journals, Newspapers

Aist, Clark S. "Pastoral Care of the Mentally Ill: A Congregational Perspective." *Journal of Pastoral Care.* 41(4) (Dec. 1987):299-310.

Anderson, Robert G. "The Assessment of Systems in Promoting Collaborative Aftercare: Religious and Mental Health Organizations in Partnership." *Journal of Pastoral Care* 39(3) (Sept. 1985): 236-248.

Armbrister, Trevor. "Return of Marie Balter." *Reader's Digest,* July 1991, 123.

Bach, Paul J. "Demon Possession and Psychopathology: A Theological Relationship." *Journal of Psychology and Theology* 7(1) (1979): 22-30.

Barrett, Katherine, and Richard Green: "Mom, Please Get Me Out!" *Ladies Home Journal,* May 1990, 98.

Brownlee, Shannon. "Alzheimer's: Is There Hope?" *U.S. News and World Report,* 12 August 1991, 40.

Byrd, Walt. "Insanity - Under Whose Law?" *The Fundamentalist Journal* 1(2) (October 1982): 38-39.

Cannon, John M. "Pastoral Care for Families of the Mentally Ill." *The Journal of Pastoral Care* 44(3) (Fall 1990): 213-221.

Eimer, Kenneth W. "The Assessment and Treatment of the Religiously Concerned Psychiatric Patient." *The Journal of Pastoral Care* 43(3) (Fall 1989): 231-241.

Erickson, Richard C., David Cutler, Victoria Brannon Cowell,and George E. Dobler. "Serving the Needs of Persons with Chronic Mental Illness: A Neglected Ministry." *The Journal of Pastoral Care* 44(2) (Summer 1990): 153-162.

Gershan, Elliot S. and Ronald O. Rieder. "Major Disorders of Mind and Brain." *Scientific American* 267 (September 1992): 126-133.

Goode, Erica E. "When Mental Illness Hits Home." *U.S. News and World Report*, 24 April 1989, 55.

Goode, Erica E. "Sick or Just Quirky?" *U.S. News and World Report*, 10 February 1992, 49.

Govig, Stewart P. "Wilderness Journal: Parental Engagement with Young Adult Mental Illness." *World and World* 9(2) (Spring, 1989): 14-20.

Hasker, William. "The Critique of Mental Illness: Conceptual and/or Ethical Crisis." *Journal of Psychology and Theology* 5(2) (1977): 110-124.

Heimstra, William L. "Do We Need Christian Mental Hospitals?" *The Reformed Review* 17(4) (1964): 25-32.

Hiltner, Seward. "Report on Mental Illness." *Pastoral Psychology* 12(114) (May 1961):49-52.

Holinger, Paul C. "Pastoral Care of the Severely Emotionally Distressed: An Overview of Potential Pastoral Roles in the Clinical Setting." *Pastoral Psychology* 29(2) (Winter 1980): 134-148.

Hyder, Quentin O. "On the Mental Health of Jesus Christ." *Journal of Psychology and Theology* 5(1) (1977): 3-12.

Isaac, Rael Jean, and Virginia C. Armat. "Hostages To Madness." *Reader's Digest*, January 1991, 92.

Isaacs, T. Craig. "The Possessive States Disorder: The Diagnosis of Demonic Possession." *Pastoral Psychology* 35(4) (1987): 263-273.

Jackson, Basil. "Psychology, Psychiatry, and the Pastor." *Bibliotheca Sacra* 132 (Jan.-March 1975): 3-15.

Johnson, Walter. "Demon Possession and Mental Illness." *Journal of the American Scientific Affiliation* 34(4) (1982): 149-154.

Klink, Thomas W. "Pastoral Problems in the Psychiatric Hospital." *The Journal of Pastoral Care* 15(1) (Spring 1961): 25-31.

Koteskey, Ronald L. "Abandoning the Psyche to Secular Treatment." *Christianity Today* 23(18) (1979): 985- 987.

Johnson, Walter. "Demon Possession and Mental Illness." *Journal of the American Scientific Affiliation* 34(4) (1982): 149-154.

Klink, Thomas W. "Pastoral Problems in the Psychiatric Hospital." *The Journal of Pastoral Care* 15(1) (Spring 1961): 25-31.

Koteskey, Ronald L. "Abandoning the Psyche to Secular Treatment." *Christianity Today* 23(18) (1979): 985- 987.

Meigs, Thomas J. "Pastoral Care Methods and Demonology in Selected Writings." *Journal of Psychology and Theology* 5(3) (Summer, 1977): 234-246.

Mowrer, O. Hobart. "The New Challenge to Our Churches and Seminaries." *Foundations* 3(4) (Oct. 1960): 335-347.

Oates, Wayne E. "New Emphases in Psychiatry and Religion: DSM-III." *Union Seminary Quarterly Review* 36(2-3) (Winter/Spring 1981): 141-147.

Olsen, Loren M. "From Embarrassment to Embrace: Ministry to the Mentally Ill." *Lexington Theological Quarterly* 27(2) (April 1992): 61-67.

"New Drug Gives Schizophrenics New Hope." *Amarillo Globe News*, 29 January 1992, Sec. A, p.1.

Peters, Frank C. "Counseling and Pastoral Training." *Bibliotheca Sacra* 126 (Oct. 1969): 291-299.

Reed, John P. "Mind/Brain in the Age of Psychopharmacology: A Crossroads for Medicine and Ministry." *The Journal of Pastoral Care* 35(1) (March 1981): 3-17.

Sall, Millard J. "A Response To 'Demon Possession and Psychopathology: A Theological Relationship.'" *Journal of Psychology and Theology* 7(1) (1979): 27- 30.

Sall, Millard J. "Demon Possession or Psychopathology? A Critical Differentiation." *Journal of Psychology and Theology* 4(4) (1976): 286-290.

Songer, Harold S. "Demon Possession and Mental Illness." *Religion in Life* 36(1967): 119-127.

Southard, Samuel. "Demonizing and Mental Illness (2): The Problem of Assessment: Los Angeles." *Pastoral Psychology* 34(4) (1986): 264-287.

Southard, Samuel and Donna. "Demonizing and Mental Illness." *East Asia Journal of Theology* (4:2) (1986): 170-183.

Southard, Samuel and Donna. "Demonizing and Mental Illness (III): Explanations and Treatment, Seoul." *Pastoral Psychology* 35(2) (Winter 1986): 132-151.

Stafford, Tim. "Franchising Hope." *Christianity Today,* 18 May 1992, 22.

"The Father of Reagan's Assailant Devotes His Life to Combating Mental Illness: Jack Hinkley Talks About Mental Health Issues and His Youngest Son, John." *Christianity Today* 14 June 1985, 42-44.

Van Gelder, David W. "A Case of Demon Possession." *Journal of Pastoral Care* 41(2) (1987): 151-161.

Virkler, Henry A., and Mary B. "Demonic Involvement In Human Life and Illness." *Journal of Psychology and Theology* 5(2) (1977): 95-101.

Williams, Patricia, William A. Williams, Robert Sommer, and Barbara Sommer. "A Survey of the California Alliance for the Mentally Ill." *Hospital and Community Psychiatry* 37(3) (March 1986): 253-256.

C. Monographs and Pamphlets

Annotated Reading List. Arlington, VA: National Alliance For the Mentally Ill, 1990.

Annotated Reading List Supplement 1991. Arlington, VA: National Alliance For the Mentally Ill, 1991.

Bouricius, Jean K. *Psychoactive Drugs and Their Effects Upon Mentally Ill Persons.* Arlington, VA: National Alliance For the Mentally Ill, 1989.

Dickens, Rex, ed. *NAMI Siblings and Adult Children's Network Annotated Book, Audio and Video Lists.* Rex Dickens, 1989. (Available from NAMI, Arlington, VA).

NAMI Religious Outreach Network Resource Materials. Arlington, VA: National Alliance For the Mentally Ill, n.d.

Papolos, Demitri. *Mood Disorders Depression and Manic Depression.* NAMI Medical Information Series. Arlington, VA: National Alliance For the Mentally Ill, n.d.

Schizophrenia. NAMI Medical Information Series. Arlington, VA: National Alliance For the Mentally Ill, n.d.

Shifrin, Jennifer. *Pathways to Partnership: An Awareness and Resource Guide on Mental Illness.* Second ed. Rabbi Jeffrey Cohen and Florence Kraft, ed. St. Louis, MO: Pathways to Promise, Interfaith Ministries and Prolonged Mental Illness, 1990.

Tardive Dyskinesia. NAMI Medical Information Series. Arlington, VA: National Alliance For the Mentally Ill, n.d.

The Experiences of Patients and Families: First Person Accounts. Reprint from Schizophrenia Bulletin and New York Times. Arlington, VA: National Alliance For The Mentally Ill, 1989.

Organizational Leaflets, Brochures, and Position Papers

"A Consumer's Guide to the Commitment Process under the Texas Mental Health Code." Austin, TX: Advocacy Inc., n.d.

"Chronic Mental Illness: A Congregational Challenge." A paper issued by the Standing Committee for Church in Society, the American Lutheran Church. Minneapolis: Augsburg Publishing House, n.d.

"Facts About Mental Illness." Austin, TX: Texas Alliance For the Mentally Ill, n.d.

"What Is Schizophrenia?" Arlington, VA: National Alliance For the Mentally Ill, n.d.

"What You Don't Know About Mental Illness Could Fill a Booklet." Falls Church, VA: The American Mental Health Fund, n.d.

E. Cassettes Audio/Video

"News From Medicine: Peace of Mind." Atlanta, GA, Cable News Network, 1988.

Waterhouse, Steven. "Many Are the Afflictions of the Righteous." *Westcliff Bible Tapes.* Amarillo, TX, 18 June 1989.

Waterhouse, Steven. "Psychology: Virtue, Voodoo or Limited Value?" *Westcliff Bible Tapes.* 8 April 1990.

Waterhouse, Steven. "The Christian Mind." Amarillo, TX, *Westcliff Bible Tapes.* 23 June 1991.

F. Unpublished Research Papers, Theses, and Dissertations

McIlroy, Charles B. "After Care for the Mentally Ill." Ph.D. diss., Western Conservative Baptist Seminary, 1986.

Oppenheimer, David. "Is the Cause of Schizophrenia Neurobio-logical or Psychosocial in Nature?" A Research paper presented to Liberty University School of Lifelong Learning. 30 June 1991.

Quinn, James B. "A Christian Perspective of Drug Therapy." Th. M. thesis, Dallas Theological Seminary, 1981.

Waterhouse, Steven. "Demons and Pastoral Care." A research paper presented to Kerby Anderson, Dallas Theological Seminary. 15 April 1991.

G. U.S. Government Documents

National Institute of Mental Health. *Caring for People With Severe Mental Disorders: A National Plan of Research to Improve Services.* DHHS Pub. No. (ADM) 91-1762. Washington, D.C.: Supt of Docs., U.S. Govt. Print. Off., 1991.

Shore, David, ed. *Schizophrenia: Questions and Answers.* Rockville, MD: National Institute of Mental Health, U.S. Department of Health and Human Services, 1986.

U.S. Department of Education. *Pocket Guide to Federal Help for Individuals with Disabilities.* Washington, D.C.: U.S. Government Printing Office, 1989.

U.S. Department of Health and Human Services, National Institute of Mental Health. reprint edition A. *National Plan for Schizophrenia Research: Panel Recommendations*, 1988.

U.S. Department of Health and Human Services, National Institute of Mental Health. *A National Plan for Schizophrenia Research: Report of the National Advisory Mental Health Council*, 1988.

U.S. Department of Health and Human Services, National Institute of Mental Health. *A Synthesis of NIMH-Funded Research Concerning Persons Who Are Homeless and Mentally Ill,* 1989.

U.S. Department of Health and Human Services, National Institute of Mental Health. *Approaching the 21st Century: Opportunities for NIMH Neuroscience Research,* 1988.

U.S. Department of Health and Human Services. *National Plan for Research on Child and Adolescent Mental Disorders,* 1990.

U.S. Department of Health and Human Services, National Institute of Mental Health. Special Report: *Schizophrenia,* 1987.

Endorsements

Strength For His People by Rev. Steven Waterhouse is a very helpful book for families of patients suffering from Schizophrenia. Having suffered with a brother who has severe Schizophrenia, he speaks from personal experience, not just theoretical or academic learning. His book can, also, be very helpful for pastors, church counselors and any deeply religious persons who are confused and uncertain how to think about mental illness in a Christian context. This book also does a nice job of separating out demon possession from mental illness, which can be very helpful since many patients with Schizophrenia and also well meaning pastors and Christian family members confuse the two conditions. Unfortunately, such confusion has often led to poor advice resulting in patients with Schizophrenia stopping their medication, leading to disaster.

I can recommend this book without hesitation to families, friends and pastors of patients with Schizophrenia and to church related counselors to help them understand and deal with mentally ill patients in a caring, loving and Christian way.

Donald H. Gent, M.D., F.A.P.A.
President, Psychiatry Section
Christian Medical and Dental Society

Strength For His People has been an invaluable tool in helping me provide educational services for the friends and relatives of people with mental illness. We can no longer ignore the spiritual questions that arise when mental illness strikes a Christian family. I would recommend *Strength For His People* to any mental health professional who works with the families or consumers of mental health services.

Melody Jenkins, M. Ed.
Director, Family and Community Education
Texas Panhandle Mental Health Authority
Texas Health and Human Services
Amarillo, Texas